Better Homes and Gardens®

CALORIE COUNTER'S
COOK BOOK

© Copyright 1983 by Meredith Corporation, Des Moines, Iowa.
All Rights Reserved. Printed in the United States of America.
Second Edition. Third Printing, 1984.
Library of Congress Catalog Card Number: 82-80530
ISBN: 0-696-00835-1

On the cover: Seafood Rolls (see recipe, page 33)

BETTER HOMES AND GARDENS® BOOKS
Editor: Gerald M. Knox
Art Director: Ernest Shelton
Managing Editor: David A. Kirchner

Food and Nutrition Editor: Doris Eby
Department Head, Cook Books: Sharyl Heiken
Senior Food Editors: Rosemary C. Hutchinson,
    Elizabeth Woolever
Senior Associate Food Editor: Sandra Granseth
Associate Food Editors: Jill Burmeister, Linda Henry,
    Julia Malloy, Alethea Sparks, Marcia Stanley,
    Diane Yanney
Recipe Development Editor: Marion Viall
Test Kitchen Director: Sharon Stilwell
Test Kitchen Home Economists: Jean Brekke,
    Kay Cargill, Marilyn Cornelius, Maryellyn Krantz,
    Marge Steenson

Associate Art Director (Managing): Randall Yontz
Associate Art Directors (Creative): Linda Ford,
    Neoma Alt West
Copy and Production Editors: Nancy Nowiszewski,
    Lamont Olson, Mary Helen Schiltz, David A. Walsh
Assistant Art Directors: Harijs Priekulis, Tom Wegner
Graphic Designers: Mike Burns, Trish Church-
    Podlasek, Alisann Dixon, Mike Eagleton, Lynda
    Haupert, Deb Miner, Lyne Neymeyer, Stan Sams,
    D. Greg Thompson, Darla Whipple, Paul Zimmerman

Editor in Chief: Neil Kuehnl
Group Editorial Services Director: Duane L. Gregg

General Manager: Fred Stines
Director of Publishing: Robert B. Nelson
Director of Retail Marketing: Jamie Martin
Director of Direct Marketing: Arthur Heydendael

CALORIE COUNTER'S COOK BOOK
Editor: Elizabeth Woolever
Copy and Production Editor: Lamont Olson
Graphic Designer: Deb Miner
Consultant: Joyce Trollope

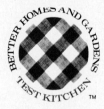

Our seal assures you that every recipe in **Calorie Counter's Cook Book** has been tested in the Better Homes and Gardens Test Kitchen. This means that each recipe is practical and reliable, and meets our high standards of taste appeal.

CONTENTS

BEFORE YOU BEGIN

Food contributes much more than calories to the diet, although calories are frequently a major concern. On the next few pages you'll find information about calories and why you need to keep track of them, as well as information on the basic nutrients necessary to a healthy diet.

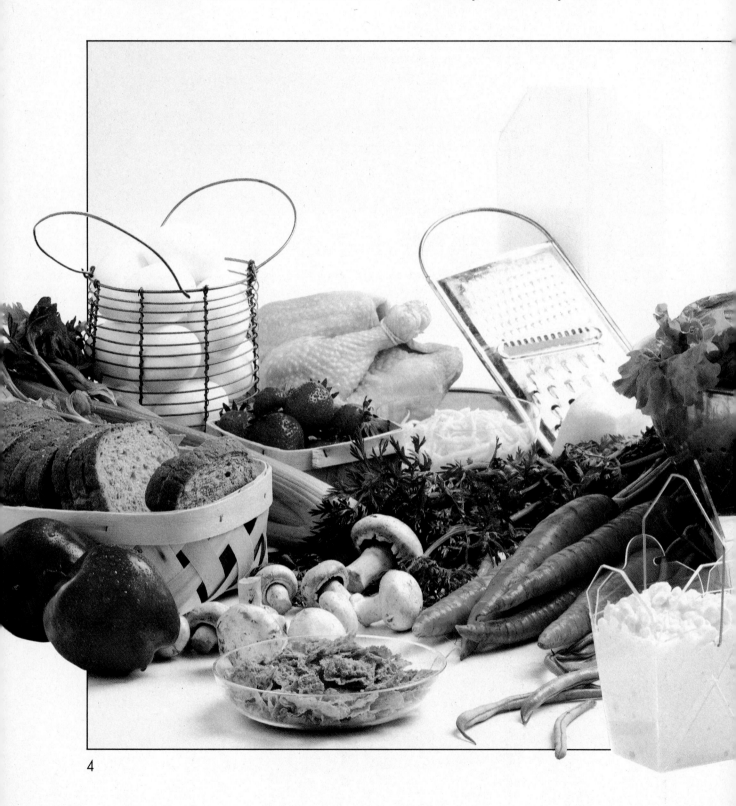

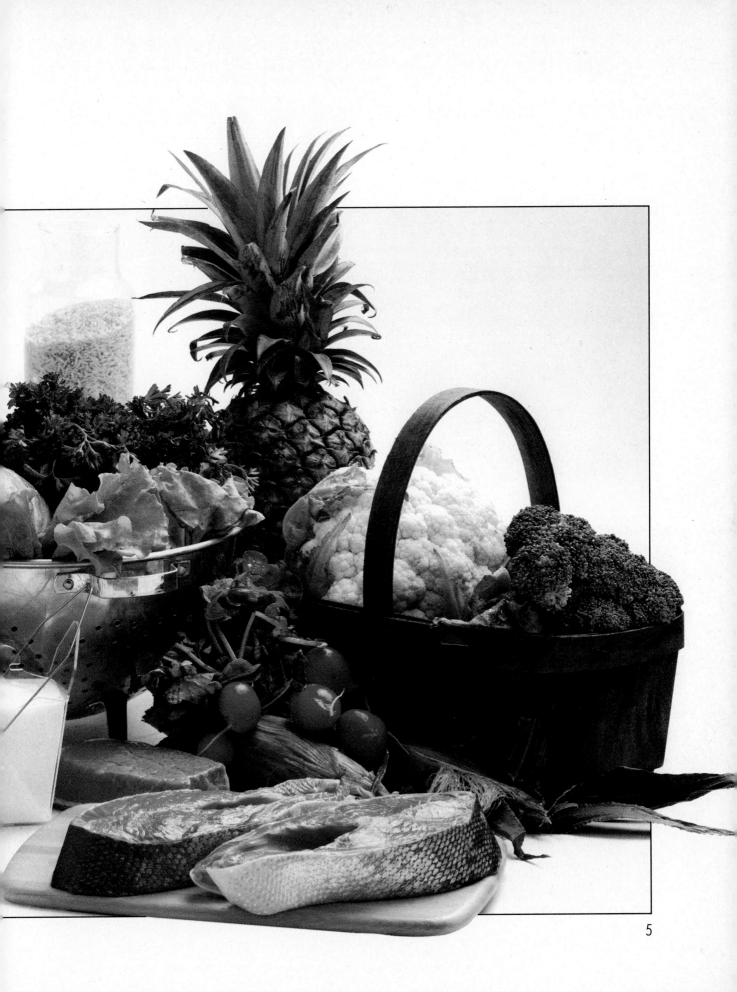

*E*ating is something most of us do a number of times each day, sometimes without stopping to consider that we need to balance the number of calories we consume with the amount of calories our body is using. Unfortunately for many Americans, this lack of balance shows. The body has an almost endless capacity for storing excess calories in the form of body fat, which keeps track of how many extra calories we eat each day even if we don't. Not only are extra pounds bothersome from a social and psychological standpoint, but they may interfere with our mobility. Research points to significant correlations between overweight and chronic diseases such as heart attack, stroke, diabetes, gallbladder disease, and certain forms of cancer.

What are calories?

A calorie is a measure of the amount of energy provided to your body by the food you eat. Regardless of whether you want to maintain your body weight or reduce it, both the calorie content of your daily food intake and the energy you expend are important.

One pound of stored body fat contains the energy equivalent of about 3,500 calories. If you want to lose weight, you will have to consume fewer calories or increase your activity to expend extra energy, or do both.

Calorie needs

How can you figure your daily calorie needs? First, you must calculate approximately how many calories your body needs each day to *maintain your current weight*. Do this by multiplying your weight by 15. (Fifteen is an average; women usually burn around 14 calories per pound and men 16 calories per pound if they are getting moderate exercise.)

To determine your daily calorie level needed to *lose weight*, subtract either 500 or 1,000 calories from the number needed to maintain your present weight. By subtracting 500 calories, you can expect a loss of about one pound per week. By subtracting 1,000 calories from your daily maintenance level, you have the lower number needed for a two-pound weight loss each week.

A word of caution: It is advisable not to follow a reducing plan that provides fewer than 1,000 calories per day. The body needs more than 40 nutrients in varying amounts each day in addition to the daily calorie requirement. It is virtually impossible to get the proper amounts of those nutrients on intakes of less than 1,000 calories, no matter how judicious you are in daily menu planning. It is also important that you check with a physician before beginning any weight-loss plan.

Exercising helps too

Exercising increases the need for energy (or calories). You must be careful not to assume that the body needs more calories because you feel "tired." In fact, most people note that increased exercise actually has the opposite effect, leaving them feeling more energetic. Another bonus for exercising is that it burns up the unwanted calories that have been stored as fat. A regular exercise program is the perfect partner for a calorie-reduced food intake.

Getting the most nutrition for your calories

In addition to calories, food provides many other nutrients. All are important to your total daily nutrition, each performing different (although interrelated) functions within the body.

PROTEIN is necessary for growth and repair of body tissue. It is needed for production of the antibodies that combat disease and for production of the enzymes and hormones that regulate body processes. Protein is found in animal products such as meat, fish, poultry, eggs, and dairy products. In addition, plants provide protein in dried beans and peas, whole grains, cereals, seeds, and nuts. The daily recommended amount of protein for adults is not difficult to attain with the average American diet. In fact, most Americans eat two to three times the amount of protein they need each day.

CARBOHYDRATES provide the body with energy. In addition, many foods that contain carbohydrates provide significant amounts of vitamins, minerals, and dietary fiber.

Carbohydrates are usually classified as either simple or complex. Simple carbohydrates are sugars and concentrated sweets. They provide calories with practically no other nutrients. For this reason, they are often called "empty calories." Complex carbohydrates or starches are found in such foods as breads, cereals, grains, rice, pasta, potatoes, and dried beans and peas. The complex carbohydrates are nutrient packed and contain important dietary fiber. In addition, when eaten plain, complex carbohydrates contain virtually no fat and are low in calories.

Dietary fiber found in complex carbohydrates is an indigestible material adding "bulk" to the diet. This "bulk" helps promote proper elimination naturally. Research points to the inclusion of dietary fiber as important in the prevention of chronic diseases such as cancer of the colon, diverticulosis, and hemorrhoids. In addition, it may reduce the need for insulin in a person with insulin-dependent diabetes mellitus.

FATS supply energy and essential fatty acids, and they play a role in the absorption of vitamins A, D, E, and K. Fats supply the largest amount of calories per gram, more than double the amount provided by a gram of protein or carbohydrates. For this reason, fat is considered "calorically dense." In other words, a small amount of fat provides a lot of calories in your diet.

Decreasing the amount of fat in your diet not only helps reduce the calories, but also helps reduce your risk of developing heart disease and certain cancers to which a large intake of fat has been linked. Gradually reduce your intake of the foods highest in fat such as oils, butter, margarine, shortening, meat, fried foods, eggs, salad dressings, nuts, baked products, and certain dairy products that are high in fat.

VITAMINS are needed in very small amounts, but vitamins are essential for multiple chemical reactions and functions in your body. Some vitamins and their importance are:

▶ *Vitamin A* helps your eyes to adapt to light and dark and maintains healthy hair, skin, and mucous membranes. Vitamin A is also necessary for growth and for reproduction. Green and yellow vegetables and fruits are the best sources.

▶ *Vitamin C* is needed for the building of bones and teeth, for healthy gums and blood vessels, and wound healing. Get vitamin C in your diet by eating citrus fruits, green leafy vegetables, strawberries, tomatoes, and potatoes.

▶ *Thiamine* is a B vitamin (B_1) which regulates appetite and digestion, maintains healthy nerves, and helps release energy from the food you eat. Thiamine is found in a variety of foods. The best sources of this vitamin are pork, peanuts, fruits, vegetables, and grains.

▶ *Riboflavin* (B_2) aids in the process of food metabolism, promotes a healthy mouth and skin, and helps cells use oxygen. Sources of riboflavin are milk, meats (variety meats in particular), eggs, cheese, and whole grain or enriched cereals and breads.

▶ *Niacin* (B_3) helps your body release energy from foods you eat along with keeping the skin, digestive system, and nervous system healthy. Niacin-rich foods are poultry, fish, cheese, and enriched or whole grains.

MINERALS are needed in minute amounts, but nonetheless are crucial to your health. Minerals form parts of body structures and stimulate the action of vitamins. Some minerals and what they do for you are:

▶ *Calcium* builds and maintains your bones and teeth. It also aids in blood clotting, muscle and nerve contraction, and rhythmic heartbeat. Calcium is found in dairy products, green vegetables, and dried beans and peas.

▶ *Iron* aids in the formation of muscle and red blood cells as well as numerous enzymes. Most foods contain iron. The best sources are meat, bran cereals, dried beans and peas, prunes, and dark green vegetables.

▶ *Sodium* helps regulate water balance in the body. Your body receives sodium primarily from salt (which is 40% sodium) and from foods processed with salt and sodium compounds. The average diet includes three to ten times more sodium than is needed. This high sodium intake may cause water retention or high blood pressure. Reducing sodium by limiting your intake of table salt and salty, processed foods is a good suggestion to follow.

▶ *Potassium* is important in fluid and electrolyte balance and muscle contraction. Potassium is found in a wide variety of foods but is especially high in fruits and vegetables.

WATER, an often forgotten nutrient, aids in digestion, regulation of proper body temperature, carrying nutrients to body cells, and removal of waste products. You should drink six to eight glasses of water every day.

▶ Variety in the diet

Eating a variety of foods each day is important, particularly when total calories are limited for the purpose of weight loss. To enable you to make wise food choices without involving laborious calculations, nutritionists have devised the Basic Five Food Groups. These groups contain foods that are similar in nutrient composition. Total servings suggested from each group are based on Recommended Dietary Allowances, so that when you choose the proper number from each group, you can be sure of obtaining all the nutrients necessary for good health.

The Recommended Dietary Allowances (RDA) are standards set by the Food and Nutrition Board of the National Research Council for optimum nutrition intake in the United States. Recommended levels of intake for calories, protein, six minerals, and ten vitamins are given for different age groups and sex classifications. Although this listing does not cover all of the nutrients known to be needed by the human body, it is assumed that when these recommendations are met, the other nutrients will be provided in adequate amounts. The RDAs are revised periodically to keep up with scientific research.

The suggested number of servings per day from each of the food groups for an adult are:
▶ Milk-Cheese Group = 2 servings
▶ Bread-Cereal Group = 4 servings
▶ Vegetable-Fruit Group = 4 servings
▶ Meat, Poultry, Fish, Nuts, and Beans Group = 2 servings (total 4 to 6 ounces)
▶ Fats, Sweets, and Alcohol Group = no serving number is recommended. Foods from this group provide calories with few, if any, additional nutrients. If you are cutting calories to lose weight, avoid foods from this group.

Note that although the nutrient composition of the foods within each food group is similar, the calories that these items contribute vary considerably. For example, one 8-ounce glass of skim milk has 88 calories and one 8-ounce glass of whole milk contains 159 calories. Although each of these servings provides similar amounts of protein, calcium, and vitamin D, the number of calories in 8 ounces of whole milk is almost double the number contained in an 8-ounce glass of skim milk.

The calorie count of individual items in each food group is an important consideration for the calorie-cutter when selecting foods. Listed on the next page are some calorie-wise suggestions from four of the Basic Five Food Groups.

► Milk-Cheese Group: Choose low-fat and skim milk, buttermilk, plain low-fat yogurt, low-fat cottage cheese, low-fat ricotta, and lower fat hard cheeses such as Monterey Jack, Farmers, or mozzarella cheese.

► Bread-Cereal Group: Whole grain or enriched breads, cereals, pasta products; popcorn; brown and enriched rice; cornmeal; oats; and barley all are nutrition-wise choices. Not only do they provide many nutrients but they are a rich source of dietary fiber. Whole grain or enriched products from this group only become calorie culprits when they contain added fat or large amounts of other ingredients, such as nuts or sugar. Examples of these include snack crackers, sweet rolls, fritters or other deep-fat fried breads, granola, and sugared cereals.

► Vegetable-Fruit Group: Choices in this group are sometimes referred to as "nutrient-dense" meaning these foods contribute substantial quantities of the nutrients we need each day without being high in calories. (The only exception is the avocado, which is high in fat and calories.) Choose unsweetened fruits—fresh, frozen, or canned. Dried fruits are fine as long as they have no sugar added. They will taste sweeter because of their more concentrated form, but beware that the serving size will seem smaller because 12 grapes and 12 raisins have the same caloric content. Raw fruits are preferred because they contain the highest amount of dietary fiber and make you feel fuller.

Vegetables can be used raw, canned, or frozen, but avoid french fried foods and those with added sauces. Fresh or frozen vegetables contain the least amount of sodium. Like fruits, raw vegetables add dietary fiber.

► Meat, Poultry, Fish, Nuts, and Beans: Because protein sources have such variable amounts of fat, the calorie range of choices within this group is large. Fish and poultry are excellent choices for calorie-conscious persons. Beef, pork, lamb, and veal are also acceptable when lean and eaten in moderation. Watch the serving size (two to three ounces cooked weight of meat) and prepare without added fats (if possible) to help control the calories. For variety in the diet, occasionally include dried beans and peas.

► Nutrition analysis of recipes

Recipes in this book have a nutrition analysis that tells you the amount of calories, protein, carbohydrates, fats, sodium, and potassium in an individual serving. The nutrition analysis also gives the percentages of the United States Recommended Daily Allowances (U.S. RDAs) for protein and certain vitamins and minerals per serving. (The U.S. RDAs are simplified and condensed RDAs used on nutrition labeling.) Use the analyses to compare nutritional values of recipes. Plan your daily menus by finding recipes that will meet your calorie and nutritional needs. For ease of comparison of recipes we have put the nutrition analyses at the beginning of the chapters.

The information for nutrition analyses of recipes comes from a computerized method using Agriculture Handbook No. 456, published by the United States Department of Agriculture, as the primary source.

To obtain the nutrition analyses, we made some assumptions:

► Garnishes and ingredients listed as optional were omitted.

► If a food was marinated and then brushed with marinade during cooking, the analysis includes the entire marinade amount.

► Dippers were not included with dip recipes unless a specific amount of vegetable is listed.

► For the main-dish meat recipes, the nutrition analyses were calculated using measurements for cooked lean meat trimmed of fat.

► When two ingredient options appear in a recipe, the nutrition analysis was calculated using the first choice of ingredients.

► When a recipe ingredient has a variable weight (such as a 2½- to 3-pound broiler-fryer chicken), the nutrition analysis was calculated using the lesser weight.

MIX AND MATCH MENUS

Menus in this chapter are calorie-counted and include a variety of foods. When using them in a day's meal plan, you need to examine your menus as a whole to see what foods are needed to round out the food groups. Look for the menus shown below on pages 14 and 18.

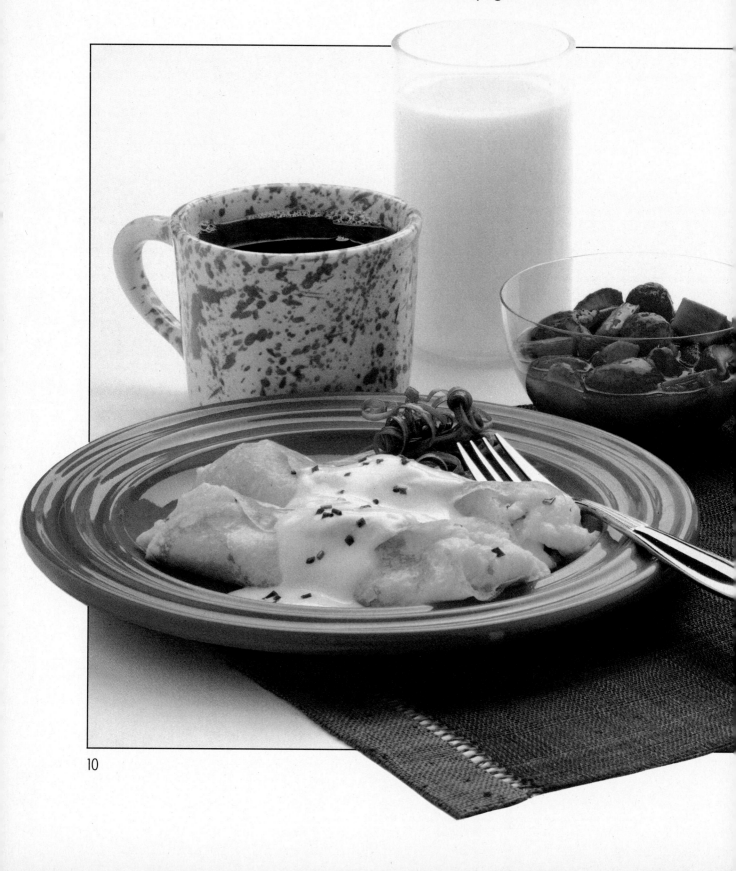

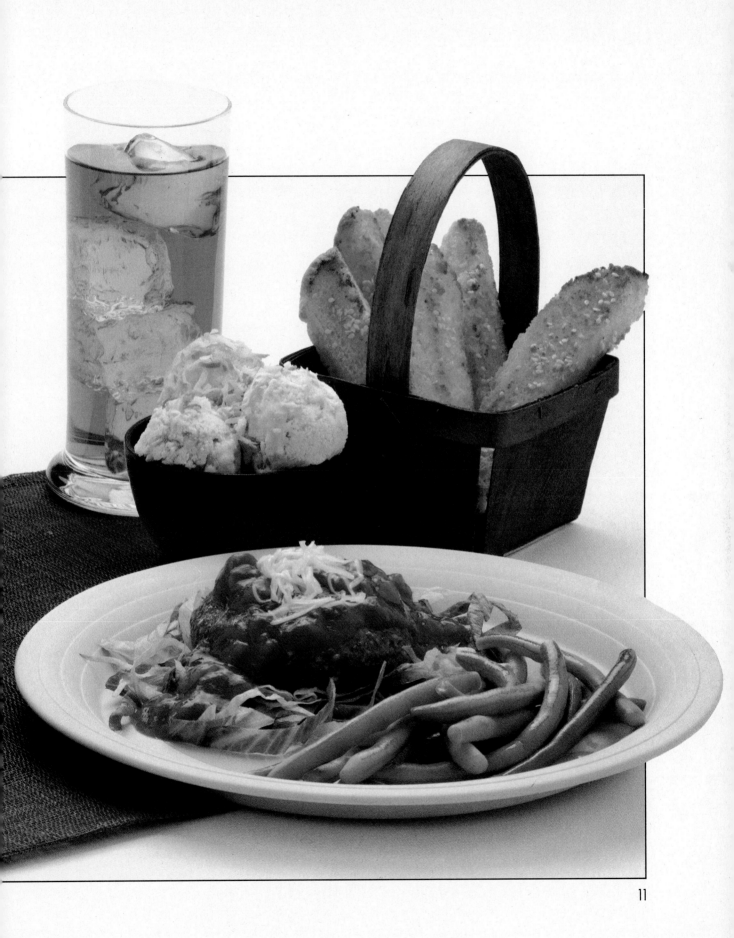

Planning calorie-conscious menus is essential to your weight control efforts. Have you found yourself needing to prepare a meal quickly with no idea how to start? Too often this situation leads to tossing together whatever you can find or eating in a fast-food restaurant. This "unplanned" eating can be the cause for so many weight control efforts to fall by the wayside.

Planning menus ahead of time when you are counting calories helps to ensure success in weight control. In addition, planning your own menus gets you involved in the decision-making and design of your weight control plan.

The basic five food groups (see pages 8 and 9) will help you plan your menus. Choosing a variety of foods from each group provides the framework for meals and snacks throughout the day.

For example, you might start designing a day's menus so that you have two servings from the Meat, Poultry, Fish, Nuts, and Beans Group by including a bean burrito at lunch and pork chop at dinner. Continue your menu planning by adding servings from the other groups. For example, the tortilla used in the burrito at lunch would count as one serving from the Bread-Cereal Group. Add and subtract servings from the other food groups until the recommended number from each group is met. Use foods in the fifth group (Fats, Sweets, and Alcohol) sparingly because they are loaded with calories and supply few nutrients.

Another approach to menu planning is to mix and match the breakfast, lunch, and dinner menus found in this chapter with each other and with your own menus. Count up the total servings for the day and compare to the basic five recommendations. Also, tally the number of calories provided by the menus and see where you stand.

If after planning your menus you find that you are still short in total servings, one way to meet the recommended number is to add them as snacks. (A piece of fresh fruit from the Vegetable-Fruit Group is an excellent choice.)

Start with the menu suggestions that follow. Then, create your own menus. When you find an especially good combination, save it to mix and match with other menus.

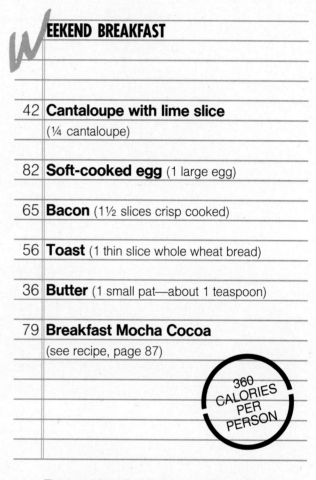

WEEKEND BREAKFAST

42 **Cantaloupe with lime slice**
(¼ cantaloupe)

82 **Soft-cooked egg** (1 large egg)

65 **Bacon** (1½ slices crisp cooked)

56 **Toast** (1 thin slice whole wheat bread)

36 **Butter** (1 small pat—about 1 teaspoon)

79 **Breakfast Mocha Cocoa**
(see recipe, page 87)

360 CALORIES PER PERSON

The breakfast shown at right doesn't take long to prepare, especially when you coordinate preparations. While the bacon bakes, prepare the beverage, soft-cook the egg, toast the bread, and cut the chilled melon.

To bake the bacon, place slices side by side on a rack in a shallow baking pan. Bake in a 400° oven for 12 to 15 minutes or till done. Before serving, thoroughly drain the bacon on paper toweling to remove excess fat.

For the soft-cooked egg, place egg in shell in a saucepan; add water to cover. Bring to boiling over high heat. Reduce heat so water is just below simmering; cover. Cook 4 to 6 minutes.

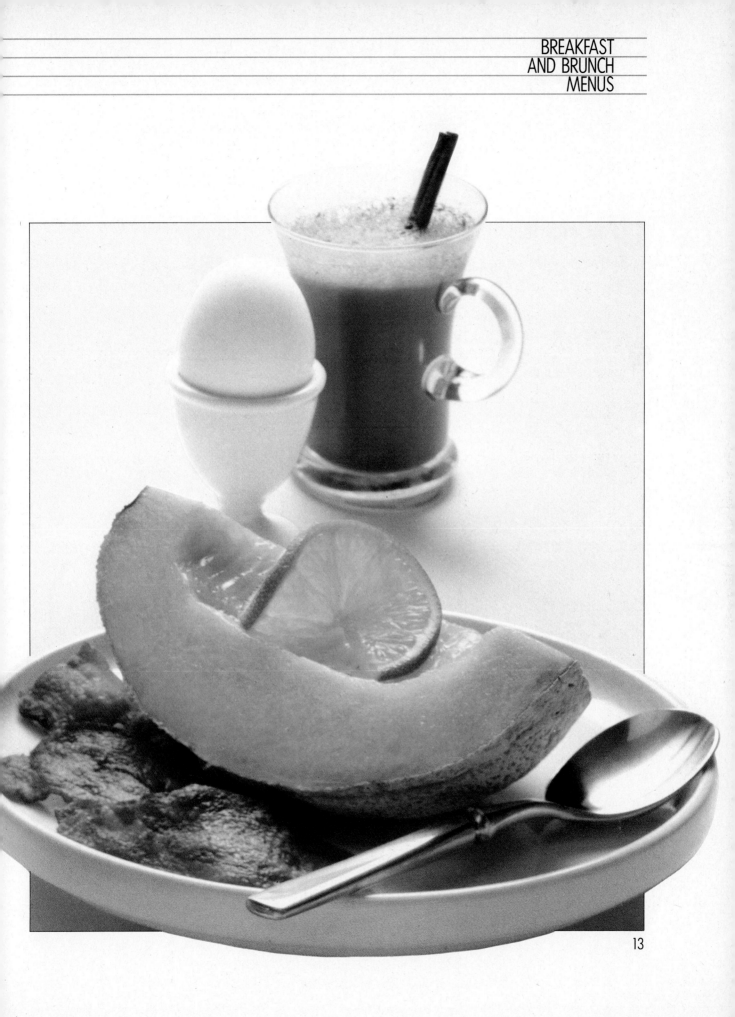

MIX AND
MATCH
MENUS

BREAKFAST
AND BRUNCH
MENUS

*B*RUNCH FOR FOUR

299	**Scrambled Egg-Filled Crepes** (see recipe, page 55)
14	**Sliced tomato** (½ of a medium tomato)
78	**Rhubarb-Strawberry Bowl** (see recipe, page 73)
88	**Skim milk** (1 cup)
2	**Coffee** (6-ounce cup)

481 CALORIES PER PERSON

The ever-popular brunch is not difficult to plan into the morning schedule if you do some of the work ahead of time. For example, in this menu, which is pictured on pages 10 and 11, you can prepare the crepes for the main dish the day before. Then fill them with the scrambled egg mixture just before you're ready to bake them. You can even prepare the crepes several weeks in advance and store them in the freezer. Be sure to thaw the crepes before adding the filling.

You can also chill the fruit mixture the day before and spoon it into dessert dishes when you are ready for the brunch. Then while the crepes bake, perk the coffee, slice the tomatoes, set the table, and pour the milk.

*Q*UICK-TO-FIX BREAKFAST

35	**Tomato juice** (6-ounce serving)
175	**Turkey and Fruit Kabobs** (see recipe, page 28)
38	**Rusk** (1, about 3½ inches in diameter)
33	**Jelly for rusk** (2 teaspoons)
66	**Skim milk** (¾ cup)

347 CALORIES PER PERSON

Try a change of pace from the cereal and toast routine in the morning. The kabobs on this menu take little time to prepare if you have cooked turkey on hand. To make the kabobs, thread turkey and fruit onto small skewers and brush with an easy-to-make sauce. The kabobs heat in the broiler with only an occasional brushing with sauce. Spread the rusk with your favorite jelly, but be sure to measure the jelly because it's one of those ingredients that adds little more than calories to the menu.

SPECIAL DAY LUNCHEON

247	**Shrimp-Swiss Soufflé** (see recipe, page 51)
100	**Vegetable Bundles with Dairy Dressing** (see recipe, page 67)
38	**Breadsticks** (two; each 7¾x¾ inches)
88	**Raspberry Ice** (see recipe, page 78)
37	**Shortbread cookie** (1)
0	**Hot tea**

510 CALORIES PER PERSON

For a special occasion, feature a soufflé for lunch. Everything else on this menu, except the hot tea, can be made ahead or purchased so you can concentrate on preparing the main dish.

Soufflés aren't that difficult to prepare, but caution must be used when handling the eggs. First, the yolks should be beaten until they flow in a thick stream from the lifted beaters. When beating the egg whites, a clean bowl (not a plastic bowl) and clean beaters must be used. The egg whites should appear moist and glossy, not dry, when they hold stiff peaks.

Serve the soufflé as soon as it is removed from the oven. Have everyone seated awaiting the entrée. Use two forks, back to back, to gently pull the soufflé into portions, then serve with a spoon.

SUMMER SALAD LUNCHEON

196	**Mandarin-Tuna-Rice Toss** (see recipe, page 35)
6	**Dill pickle spears** (2)
2	**Radishes** (2 medium)
119	**Cloverleaf roll** (one; 2½x2 inches)
36	**Butter** (1 small pat—about 1 teaspoon)
127	**Honey Buttermilk Ice Cream** (see recipe, page 79)
0	**Iced tea**

486 CALORIES PER PERSON

When the temperature soars and you don't feel like cooking a hot meal, fix a salad for lunch. Add some crisp pickle spears, radishes, and a warm roll (homemade or from the bakery). Use butter sparingly—that's where calories are added if you're not careful. Serve a cool glass of iced tea with the meal.

For dessert, crank up the ice cream freezer and turn out some calorie-counted homemade ice cream. If you can afford a few extra calories, serve the homemade ice cream with a few sliced fresh strawberries.

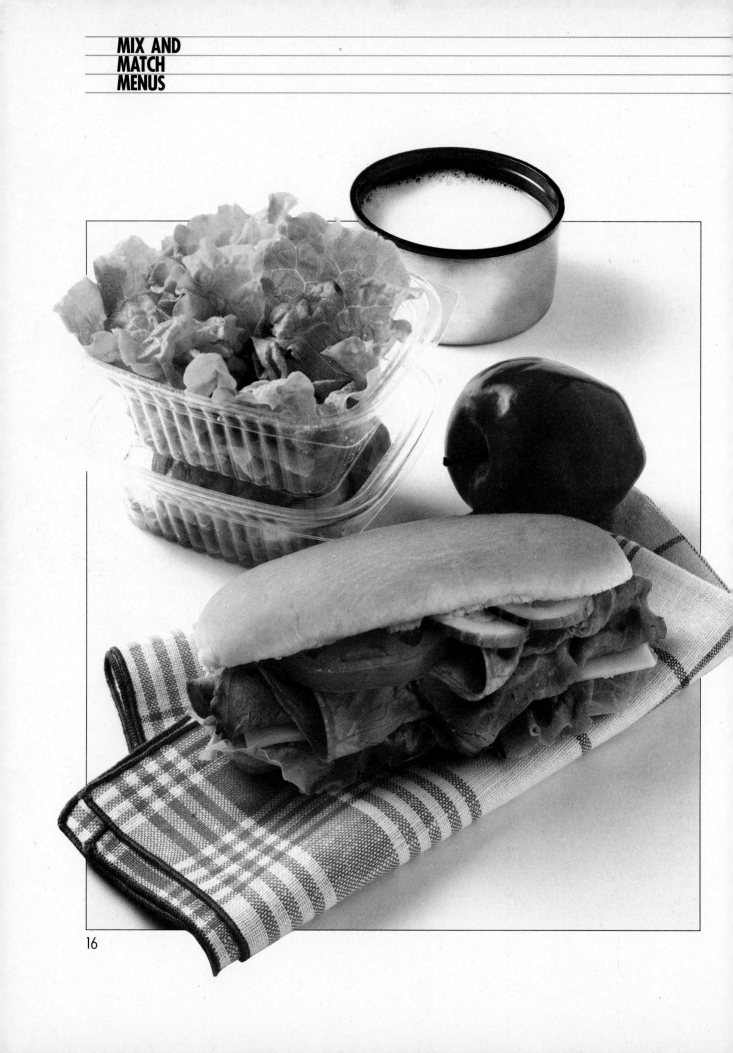

ℬROWN BAGGER'S LUNCH

294 **Garden Sandwich** (see recipe, page 40)

12 **Carrot sticks** (6 to 8 strips—about 1 ounce)

80 **Apple** (1 medium)

88 **Skim milk** (1 cup)

474
CALORIES
PER
PERSON

When you're counting calories to maintain or lose weight, packing a nutritious, interesting lunch can be a challange. The sandwich pictured at left is just one idea that may spark some other tasty sandwich possibilities. Start with some leftover beef rump roast that is trimmed of fat and thinly sliced. Stack it on a frankfurter bun with some mozzarella cheese and wrap tightly. Pack the lettuce in a plastic bag or container and pack a mixture of the tomato, cucumber, and salad dressing in a tightly covered container. Assemble the sandwich just before you're ready to eat.

Substitute another fruit for the apple if desired. Select fresh fruit or juice-pack canned fruit.

𝒮OUP AND SANDWICH LUNCH

42 **Blender Herbed Tomato Soup**
(see recipe, page 63)

260 **Ham-and-Eggers** (see recipe, page 36)

22 **Bread-and-butter pickle slices** (4)

78 **Citrus Special** (see recipe, page 76)

88 **Skim milk** (1 cup)

490
CALORIES
PER
PERSON

On a cool day a bowl of hot soup and a toasty sandwich make a good combination. Quickly whirl the tomato soup in the blender, then heat the soup while preparing the sandwich under the broiler. An open-face sandwich, such as this one, is a good calorie-cutter because it's made with only one slice of bread. Add a few pickle slices to the plate to round out the menu.

To end the meal, serve a dessert made with orange and grapefruit sections and a sliced banana. Add the topping just before serving.

If you prefer to drink whole or low-fat milk with lunch instead of skim milk, remember to add extra calories. One cup of whole milk (3.5% milk fat) has 159 calories and one cup of low-fat milk (2% milk fat) has 145 calories.

*F*AMILY-PLEASING SUPPER

273 **Diet Taco Burgers** (see recipe, page 40)

16 **Cooked green beans** (½ cup)

119 **Quick Garlic Sticks** (2 sticks)

(see recipe, page 69)

105 **Banana Freeze** (see recipe, page 78)

0 **Iced tea**

513 CALORIES PER PERSON

*G*REEK DINNER

219 **Low-Cal Moussaka** (see recipe, page 40)

24 **Cooked carrot slices** (½ cup)

74 **Calorie-Trimmed Greek Salad**

(see recipe, page 59)

78 **Hard roll** (1 roll—3¾x2½x1¾ inches)

36 **Butter** (1 small pat—about 1 teaspoon)

130 **Lemon sherbet** (½ cup)

2 **Coffee** (6-ounce cup)

563 CALORIES PER PERSON

When tacos won't fit into your calorie-counted meals, try this diet variation, which uses a bed of coarsely shredded lettuce as the base instead of a taco shell. The beef patties are broiled or grilled over charcoal so all the extra fat can drain away. Add some green beans, either cut up or whole, to the dinner plate and the quick-to-fix bread. You'll find that the easy breadsticks stretch two frankfurter buns into four servings.

Dessert is an icy mixture made with buttermilk, mashed banana, and whipped topping. Make it several hours ahead or even the night before to allow plenty of time to freeze till firm. To serve, splurge a little and sprinkle scoops of the frozen dessert with toasted coconut. This meal is pictured on pages 10 and 11.

Plan dinner with a foreign flair. The main dish, moussaka, is an interesting casserole that makes good use of ground lamb and eggplant. Bake the casserole for 15 to 20 minutes while you cook the carrots and toss the salad together. Interesting salad ingredients include the greens (romaine and escarole), crumbled feta cheese, and sliced ripe olives. Chill the dressing ahead of time. To add crispy texture to the meal, serve a small hard roll and a small pat of butter for the roll. Dessert is simple—sherbet from the grocery store. If you can afford the extra calories, accompany the sherbet with a sugar cookie.

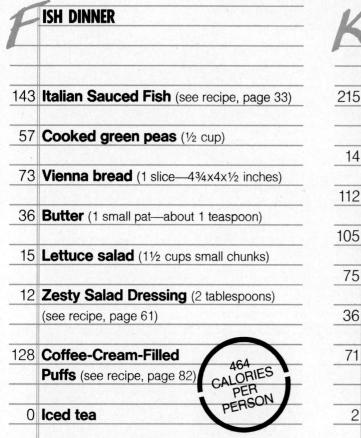

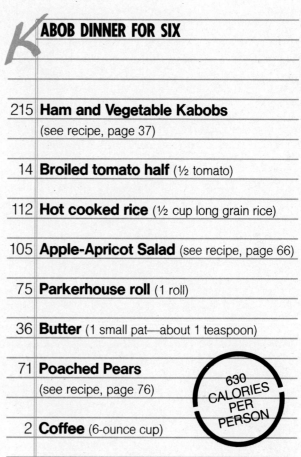

FISH DINNER

143	**Italian Sauced Fish** (see recipe, page 33)
57	**Cooked green peas** (½ cup)
73	**Vienna bread** (1 slice—4¾x4x½ inches)
36	**Butter** (1 small pat—about 1 teaspoon)
15	**Lettuce salad** (1½ cups small chunks)
12	**Zesty Salad Dressing** (2 tablespoons) (see recipe, page 61)
128	**Coffee-Cream-Filled Puffs** (see recipe, page 82)
0	**Iced tea**

464 CALORIES PER PERSON

KABOB DINNER FOR SIX

215	**Ham and Vegetable Kabobs** (see recipe, page 37)
14	**Broiled tomato half** (½ tomato)
112	**Hot cooked rice** (½ cup long grain rice)
105	**Apple-Apricot Salad** (see recipe, page 66)
75	**Parkerhouse roll** (1 roll)
36	**Butter** (1 small pat—about 1 teaspoon)
71	**Poached Pears** (see recipe, page 76)
2	**Coffee** (6-ounce cup)

630 CALORIES PER PERSON

On your next trip to the grocery store purchase a package of frozen flounder fillets, meatless spaghetti sauce, and some shredded mozzarella cheese. These are the main ingredients for the entrée featured in this menu.

The cooked salad dressing is flavored with dill, basil, garlic, and catsup and should be made ahead so it has plenty of time to chill. If desired, use a variety of salad greens instead of lettuce.

Bake a batch of cream puffs. Stash four of them in the freezer and use the remaining four for dessert. The cream puff filling consists of four ingredients—an egg white, which you beat with cream of tartar and coffee crystals, and some frozen whipped dessert topping, which is folded into the egg white.

Advance preparation for this meal includes marinating the meat and precooked vegetables for the kabobs in the refrigerator and chilling the gelatin salad. When you're ready to begin dinner preparation, start by poaching the fresh pear halves. Treat the pears with ascorbic acid color keeper to prevent them from turning brown.

Then, cook the rice, broil the kabobs and tomato halves, unmold the salads, and perk the coffee. If you wish, sprinkle the cooked rice with snipped parsley and garnish the poached pears with a fresh mint sprig to add color to this meal for six.

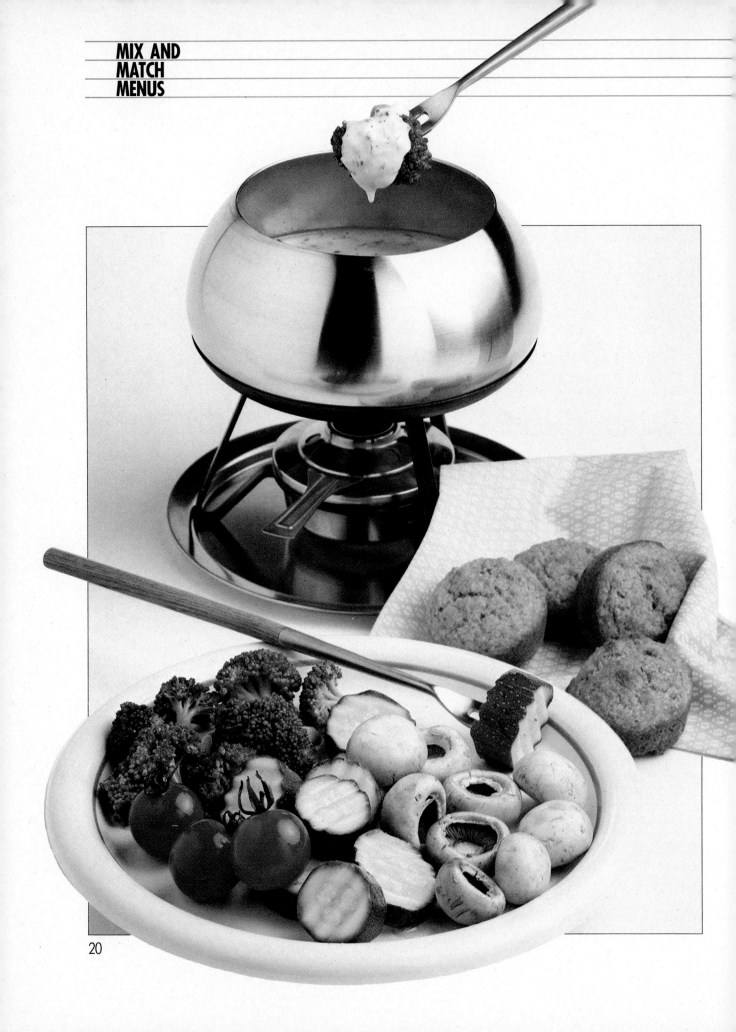

F ONDUE SUPPER

213 **Herbed Cottage-Swiss Fondue**

(see recipe, page 53)

94 **Orange-Wheat Muffins** (1 muffin)

(see recipe, page 69)

81 **Gelatin salad with banana and grapes**

(½ cup)

75 **Apple-Berry Dessert** (see recipe, page 75)

88 **Skim milk** (1 cup)

551 CALORIES PER PERSON

D INNER FOR TWO

287 **Stuffed Cabbage Rolls for Two**

(see recipe, page 41)

24 **Cooked carrot slices** (½ cup)

102 **Toasted French bread**

(1 slice—5x2½x1 inches)

36 **Butter** (1 small pat—about 1 teaspoon)

67 **Blueberry-Melon Salad** (see recipe,

page 59)

79 **Four-Fruit Ice**

(see recipe, page 73)

2 **Coffee** (6-ounce cup)

597 CALORIES PER PERSON

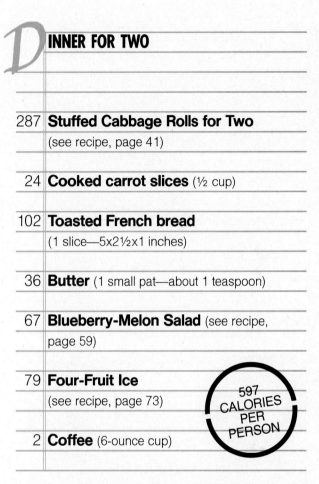

Fondue meals such as the one pictured at left are fun for the whole family, and this nutritious cheese fondue is one way for the youngsters to enjoy their vegetables. Prepare a simple gelatin salad ahead and chill it. Next, prepare and bake the muffins. Because the diet menu allows only one muffin per person, freeze the rest of the muffins for another meal. Remember to reheat the muffins before serving.

Dessert is a snap to make because all you do is toss apples and blueberries or raspberries with a honey-sweetened pineapple juice mixture.

Cooking for two people is difficult enough without having to watch the calories as well. The cabbage rolls planned for this dinner menu are a good choice to please even the fussiest of appetites, and a serving of the cabbage seems generous—two rolls per person. If you don't have the cooked rice on hand for the cabbage rolls, you'll have to prepare some according to package directions. Refrigerate the leftover rice for another meal.

The melon-berry salad sports a dressing of fruit-flavored yogurt. Then a little shredded orange peel is sprinkled atop. Dessert is another fruitful delight that can be on hand in the freezer. Serve some of it for this meal and save the rest for other meals. You'll find that the dessert servings also seem large for a diet portion.

I TALIAN-STYLE DINNER

270 **Chicken-Sauced Spaghetti**

(see recipe, page 45)

36 **Cooked broccoli** (1 small stalk)

15 **Lettuce salad** (1½ cups small chunks)

22 **Spicy Salad Dressing** (2 tablespoons)

(see recipe, page 62)

125 **Carob Tortoni** (see recipe, page 78)

0 **Hot tea**

468 CALORIES PER PERSON

C ANDLELIGHT DINNER FOR SIX

221 **Elegant Chicken Breasts**

(see recipe, page 45)

116 **Hot cooked brown rice** (½ cup long grain)

61 **Peas and Onions** (see recipe, page 64)

36 **Spinach-Mushroom Salad**

(see recipe, page 59)

123 **Orange Cheesecake Dessert**

(see recipe, page 79)

2 **Coffee** (6-ounce cup)

559 CALORIES PER PERSON

Get out the red and white checkered tablecloth and plan an Italian meal, even though you are on a diet. Did you ever think that spaghetti could be planned into your diet meals? The spaghetti sauce for this menu is made with cooked chicken instead of the more familiar sausage or ground beef. Or you can substitute cooked turkey for the chicken in the spaghetti sauce.

The salad dressing is remindful of an Italian-style dressing and is served over lettuce. If you want to add a few crispy croutons to the salad, add the additional calories, too.

For dessert, serve a mock tortoni. The recipe in this menu is flavored with carob powder with a few almonds and maraschino cherries added for color and texture.

Although your reducing diet probably doesn't play a major role when planning a special occasion meal, the menu pictured at right allows you to stick with a low-calorie diet. To begin meal preparations, start with the cheesecake dessert. While dessert is chilling in stemmed glasses, marinate fresh mushrooms for the salad in low-cal salad dressing. Then, begin by cooking the brown rice. Next, prepare the main dish. While the chicken breasts simmer in a pineapple juice mixture, cook the peas, toss the salad together, and prepare any garnishes. Set the table, light the candles, and you're ready to serve.

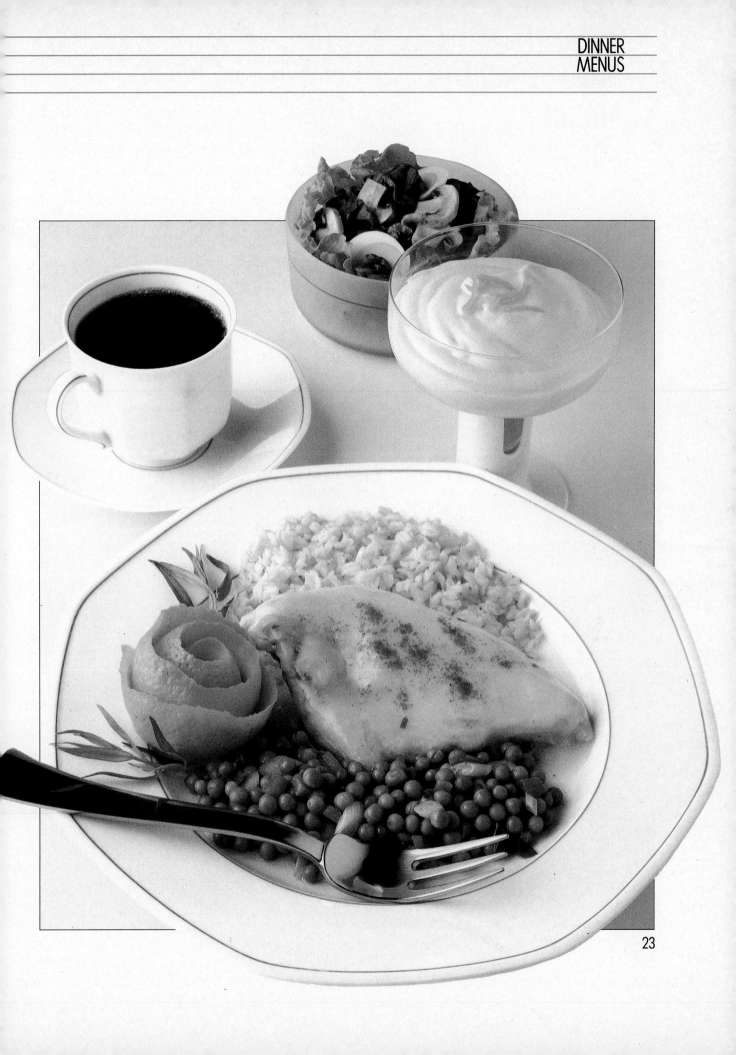

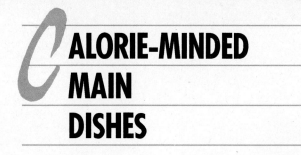

CALORIE-MINDED MAIN DISHES

Plan the rest of your calorie-counted menu around one of the nutritious and tasty main dishes in this section. Possible suggestions shown here include: Whole Wheat Meatless Pizza, Chicken and Grapes, Stir-Fried Gazpacho Salad, or Seafood Rolls (see index for recipe page numbers).

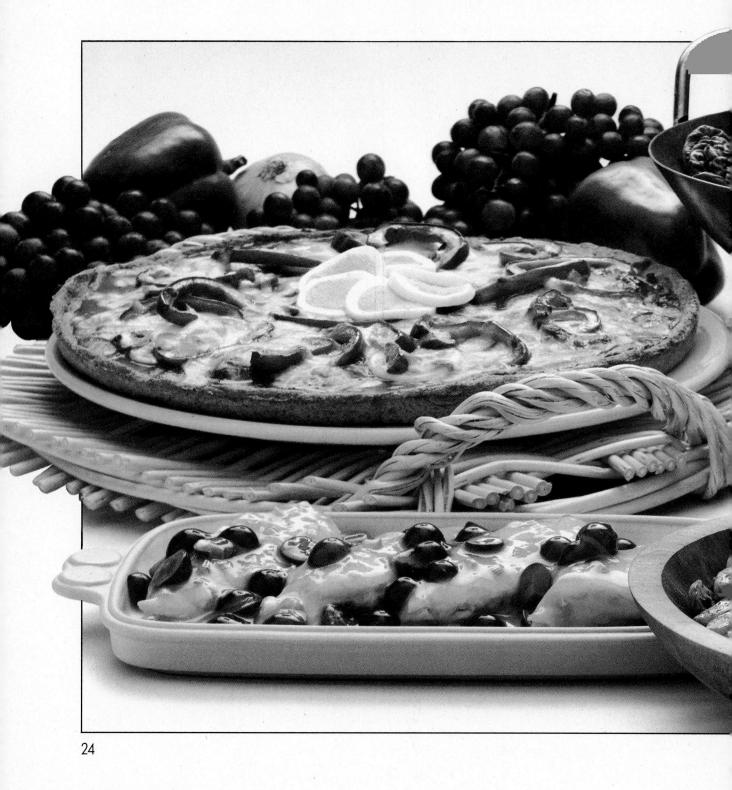

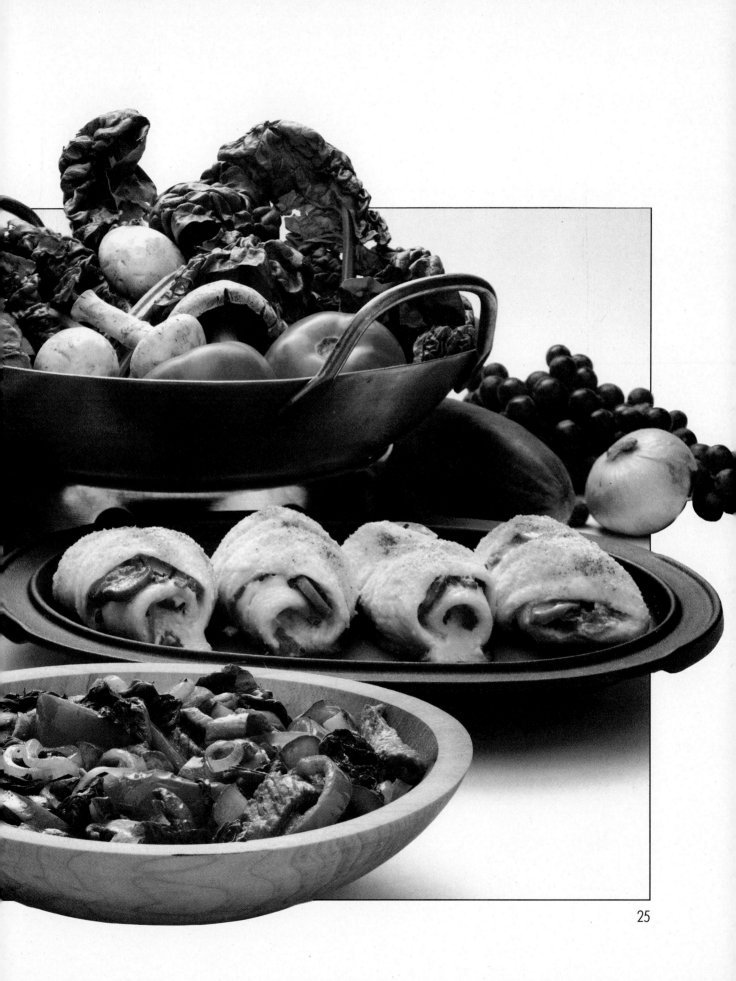

CALORIES PER SERVING		PROTEIN (g)	CARBOHYDRATE (g)	FAT (g)	SODIUM (mg)	POTASSIUM (mg)	PROTEIN	VITAMIN A	VITAMIN C	THIAMINE	RIBOFLAVIN	NIACIN	CALCIUM	IRON
		Per Serving					Percent U.S. RDA Per Serving							
	Eggs and Cheese													
294	Bean-Filled Omelet (p. 53)	22	16	16	758	432	34	32	17	13	37	2	36	17
213	Herbed Cottage-Swiss Fondue (p. 53)	20	14	9	593	622	31	60	150	12	34	12	42	10
263	Macaroni-Cheese Puff (p. 53)	17	18	14	680	237	25	22	21	12	26	5	36	9
290	Potato and Spinach Skillet (p. 54)	20	23	13	777	771	31	84	84	17	27	10	21	20
299	Scrambled Egg-Filled Crepes (p. 55)	21	19	15	687	329	33	28	3	16	36	4	26	17
249	Shirred Eggs Deluxe (p. 54)	17	2	19	262	190	26	26	0	10	24	4	12	15
270	Whole Wheat Meatless Pizza (p. 54)	17	27	11	848	197	26	26	34	19	19	12	24	13
	Fish and Seafood													
210	Baked Clams and Mushrooms (p. 50)	19	12	9	739	370	30	50	9	5	21	8	35	18
230	Baked Fish Steaks (p. 51)	25	4	13	118	600	39	22	9	7	9	48	7	5
244	Cottage Cheese-Tuna Sandwiches (p. 48)	29	18	7	623	452	45	12	23	10	19	37	24	13
137	Easy Herbed Fish (p. 35)	17	2	6	114	454	27	1	14	6	4	10	8	6
143	Italian Sauced Fish (p. 33)	22	5	4	465	438	33	2	5	5	6	10	19	7
196	Mandarin-Tuna-Rice Toss (p. 35)	22	23	1	327	456	34	9	41	11	11	48	10	11
194	Orange Halibut Steaks (p. 33)	24	4	10	195	585	37	13	31	7	5	48	2	5
212	Salmon Dolmas (p. 49)	19	13	9	693	420	29	8	37	7	16	27	28	7
161	Salmon-Stuffed Tomatoes (p. 34)	20	10	5	513	679	30	27	78	9	16	30	18	8
181	Scallop Toss (p. 35)	23	8	7	394	556	35	49	26	9	14	6	26	19
156	Seafood Rolls (p. 33)	22	4	5	465	470	34	6	7	6	12	12	23	8
255	Shrimp Newburg (p. 50)	18	23	9	490	326	28	11	4	12	18	14	20	12
134	Shrimp-Stuffed Tomatoes (p. 34)	18	13	1	156	581	28	34	83	9	7	13	11	17
247	Shrimp-Swiss Soufflé (p. 51)	20	7	15	535	191	30	21	5	6	20	4	32	11
257	Shrimp Thermidor Bake (p. 50)	26	13	10	743	218	39	14	8	4	9	9	23	17
228	Tuna and Cheese Wafflewiches (p. 48)	19	17	9	365	310	29	13	12	8	11	35	8	8
160	Tuna-Lettuce Bundles (p. 33)	29	7	2	104	584	44	23	24	6	13	63	12	14
269	Tuna-Mac Casserole (p. 49)	18	32	7	638	346	28	10	13	21	24	22	30	9
264	Tuna-Stuffed Potatoes (p. 48)	21	35	5	349	970	32	7	74	13	12	45	14	12
93	Vegetable-Fish Bake (p. 35)	18	3	1	138	586	27	6	41	7	9	14	8	7
279	Wine-Poached Halibut (p. 48)	32	3	13	229	792	49	15	7	8	9	65	3	8
	Meat													
253	Basic Meat Loaf (p. 39)	19	10	15	443	251	29	5	4	9	12	21	3	15
238	Bell Peppers with Eggplant Stuffing (p. 42)	19	9	14	346	477	29	13	168	12	16	20	5	18
237	Broiled Liver with Mushrooms (p. 43)	25	7	12	228	460	38	541	52	14	208	72	1	66
138	Deviled Steak (p. 32)	16	1	7	92	197	25	4	3	3	8	16	1	11
273	Diet Taco Burgers (p. 40)	21	10	17	436	552	33	23	36	16	19	22	10	20

CALORIES PER SERVING		PROTEIN (g)	CARBOHYDRATE (g)	FAT (g)	SODIUM (mg)	POTASSIUM (mg)	PROTEIN	VITAMIN A	VITAMIN C	THIAMINE	RIBOFLAVIN	NIACIN	CALCIUM	IRON
		Per Serving					Percent U.S. RDA Per Serving							
253	Elegant Veal (p. 39)	28	5	14	412	461	43	17	39	12	19	24	10	21
294	Garden Sandwich (p. 40)	22	31	10	436	630	33	29	59	20	19	23	17	20
279	Ham and Bulgur Skillet (p. 36)	17	37	7	548	354	26	13	14	28	13	21	5	20
208	Ham and Cheese Medley (p.36)	20	17	7	654	427	30	10	16	22	20	10	22	12
260	Ham-and-Eggers (p. 36)	20	14	14	615	229	31	13	2	14	17	7	27	14
215	Ham and Vegetable Kabobs (p. 37)	21	8	11	720	502	32	85	73	34	14	20	3	18
166	Italian Veal Steak (p. 32)	17	2	9	242	309	27	11	18	5	10	19	1	13
229	Lemon-Sauced Veal Meatballs (p. 43)	22	10	10	451	284	34	8	13	9	22	21	10	16
219	Low-Cal Moussaka (p. 40)	18	10	12	551	508	28	21	27	12	21	19	9	13
143	Oven-Style Swiss Steak (p. 32)	22	3	4	509	252	33	5	4	5	13	23	1	15
224	Pineapple Pork Chops (p. 37)	18	14	11	222	329	27	1	15	48	12	20	3	14
247	Pork Chops Italiano (p. 37)	25	2	14	64	325	39	0	5	62	16	28	2	19
269	Reuben Meat Loaf (p. 42)	20	5	18	578	233	31	6	5	6	13	18	15	14
243	Stir-Fried Gazpacho Salad (p. 41)	25	12	11	416	985	39	105	119	15	35	36	9	31
287	Stuffed Cabbage Rolls for Two (p. 41)	20	19	15	817	463	31	19	76	19	18	22	7	20
250	Stuffed Peppers (p. 39)	19	16	13	429	614	30	25	368	15	22	20	19	17
212	Stuffed Steaks (p. 43)	28	11	6	640	498	42	43	48	7	14	27	4	20
258	Tangerine Broiled Ham (p. 36)	29	11	10	1051	496	45	6	55	48	17	27	4	22
180	Teriyaki Marinated Steak (p.31)	22	9	4	319	413	34	6	65	8	12	22	3	18
170	Veal Chop Suey (p. 31)	18	10	7	832	389	27	5	18	12	17	23	4	18
184	Veal Patties Parmesan (p. 32)	19	4	10	353	155	29	7	2	6	14	20	6	14
	Poultry													
244	Chicken and Apples (p. 44)	28	16	7	126	151	44	20	9	6	14	54	3	12
185	Chicken and Grapes (p. 28)	28	9	3	121	108	44	5	29	7	14	54	2	10
183	Chicken and Peaches (p. 28)	25	14	3	332	286	38	12	57	9	16	49	4	11
219	Chicken and Pineapple Curry (p. 45)	30	7	8	202	174	46	31	13	11	36	46	3	19
275	Chicken-Beef Kabobs (p. 44)	35	17	7	406	546	54	8	46	11	28	50	16	19
197	Chicken-Romaine Salad (p. 28)	24	14	5	303	630	38	48	42	8	15	34	13	17
270	Chicken-Sauced Spaghetti (p. 45)	26	32	4	414	644	39	76	36	16	15	40	4	18
168	Easy Chicken and Rice Bake (p. 29)	20	13	4	267	409	31	11	23	11	18	25	14	9
221	Elegant Chicken Breasts (p. 45)	37	6	4	178	47	58	3	5	7	17	71	3	13
299	Minted Chicken-Grapefruit Salad (p. 47)	21	36	9	154	594	32	11	132	8	10	33	7	9
238	Pepper Chicken and Sprouts (p. 44)	26	15	9	305	519	40	16	139	17	23	43	5	17
185	Pineapple-Glazed Chicken (p. 29)	24	6	6	179	65	37	20	10	8	29	36	2	15
231	Spicy Tomato Chicken for Two (p. 45)	29	7	9	348	228	45	18	21	8	15	56	3	14
175	Turkey and Fruit Kabobs (p. 28)	19	17	4	76	410	29	5	72	7	9	24	3	8
255	Turkey-Fruit Salad (p. 47)	24	23	8	213	655	37	9	101	10	15	31	8	13

185 CHICKEN AND GRAPES

Pictured on pages 24 and 25—

2 whole medium chicken breasts
   (1½ pounds total), skinned, halved
   lengthwise, and boned
½ teaspoon finely shredded orange peel
½ cup orange juice
1 teaspoon instant chicken bouillon granules
2 tablespoons chopped green onion
1 tablespoon cornstarch
½ cup halved and seeded Tokay grapes
   Paprika

Arrange chicken in a 10x6x2-inch baking dish. Set peel aside. In saucepan heat orange juice; dissolve bouillon in hot orange juice. Stir in orange peel, green onion, and dash *pepper*. Pour over chicken. Cover with foil; bake in a 350° oven for 40 to 50 minutes or till tender. Transfer chicken to a warm platter. Strain pan juices, reserving *¾ cup* for sauce. In saucepan stir together cornstarch and 2 tablespoons *cold water;* stir in reserved pan juices. Cook and stir till thickened and bubbly; cook and stir 2 minutes more. Stir in grapes; heat through. To serve, spoon sauce over chicken; sprinkle with paprika. Serves 4.

183 CHICKEN AND PEACHES

1 8-ounce can low-calorie peach slices
   (water pack)
1¼ pounds chicken breasts, skinned, halved
   lengthwise, and boned
¾ cup orange juice
4 teaspoons cornstarch
1 tablespoon soy sauce
¼ teaspoon ground ginger
1½ cups coarsely chopped zucchini

Drain peaches, reserving liquid. Cut chicken into 1-inch pieces. In saucepan simmer chicken in peach liquid, covered, about 6 minutes or till done. Stir orange juice into cornstarch. Stir in soy and ginger. Add to saucepan. Stir in zucchini. Cook and stir till bubbly and zucchini is crisp-tender. Stir in peaches; heat through. Serves 4.

197 CHICKEN-ROMAINE SALAD

1 head romaine, torn into bite-size pieces
   (8 cups)
2 cups cubed cooked chicken
2 tablespoons grated Parmesan cheese
½ cup Spicy Salad Dressing
   (see recipe, page 62)
1 tablespoon tarragon vinegar
½ teaspoon dry mustard
¼ teaspoon Worcestershire sauce
¾ cup croutons
1 small tomato, cut into wedges

In bowl combine romaine, chicken, and Parmesan. Combine Spicy Salad Dressing, vinegar, mustard, and Worcestershire. Pour mixture over salad; add croutons and tomato wedges. Toss lightly to coat with dressing. Serves 4.

175 TURKEY AND FRUIT KABOBS

You can use either boneless turkey roast or a large piece of turkey breast meat for the cubes—

8 ounces cooked turkey, cut into 1-inch cubes
   (1½ cups)
1 large seedless orange, peeled and cut
   into 16 chunks
1 firm pear, cut into 8 wedges and each wedge
   halved crosswise
1 teaspoon cornstarch
1 teaspoon brown sugar
⅛ teaspoon ground ginger
   Dash ground cloves
½ cup orange juice

Thread turkey and fruit onto eight 6-inch skewers. In small saucepan combine cornstarch, brown sugar, and spices. Stir in orange juice. Cook and stir till thickened and bubbly. Cook and stir 1 to 2 minutes longer. Brush sauce over fruit and turkey. Place on rack of unheated broiler pan. Broil about 5 inches from heat for 10 to 15 minutes or till meat and fruit are hot and well glazed. Turn and brush occasionally with sauce. Brush with sauce just before serving. Pass remaining sauce. Serves 4.

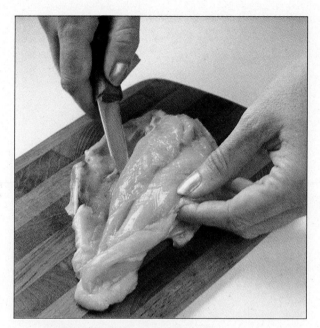

▲ BONING CHICKEN BREASTS

Chicken breasts are good for dieters, especially when they're cooked without the skin. You'll notice that some recipes call for chicken breasts that have been skinned, halved lengthwise, and boned. To do this, start by pulling the skin of the chicken breast away from the meat; discard the skin. Next, cut the chicken breast in half lengthwise.

Hold the chicken breast half with bone side down on a cutting board. Starting from the breastbone side, use a sharp knife to begin cutting meat away from the bone as shown. Cut as close to the bone as possible, using a sawing motion and pressing the flat side of the knife blade against the rib bones. With the other hand, gently pull the meat away from the rib bones of the chicken breast.

168 EASY CHICKEN AND RICE BAKE

- 1 10-ounce package frozen cut asparagus
- 2 tablespoons grated Parmesan cheese
- 2 cups cubed cooked chicken *or* turkey
- 1 cup cold cooked rice
- ¾ cup plain low-fat yogurt
- 2 tablespoons all-purpose flour
- 1 cup skim milk
- 1 teaspoon instant chicken bouillon granules
- ¼ teaspoon dried sage, crushed
- 1 tablespoon snipped parsley
- 2 tablespoons grated Parmesan cheese

Cook asparagus according to package directions; drain. Place in an 8x8x2-inch baking dish. Sprinkle with 2 tablespoons Parmesan; top with chicken or turkey. Spoon rice over all. Set aside. In saucepan stir together the yogurt and flour; stir in milk, bouillon granules, and sage. Cook and stir till thickened and bubbly. Stir in parsley. (Sauce may have a slightly grainy appearance.) Pour sauce over chicken and rice. Sprinkle with 2 tablespoons Parmesan. Bake, uncovered, in a 400° oven for 18 to 20 minutes. Serves 6.

185 PINEAPPLE-GLAZED CHICKEN

- 1 2½- to 3-pound broiler-fryer chicken, cut up and skin removed
- 1 8-ounce can crushed pineapple (juice pack)
- 1 teaspoon minced dried onion
- 2 tablespoons orange juice
- 2 teaspoons cornstarch
  Dash ground ginger

Arrange chicken in a 13x9x2-inch baking pan. Combine *undrained* pineapple, onion, and ½ teaspoon *salt*; spoon over chicken. Bake, uncovered, in a 375° oven for 50 to 60 minutes or till done; baste occasionally with pineapple mixture. Remove chicken and pineapple to platter; keep warm. Skim fat from pan juices. In saucepan combine orange juice, cornstarch, and ginger. Add about ½ cup pan juices. Cook and stir till thickened and bubbly. Cook and stir 2 minutes more. Spoon over chicken. Makes 6 servings.

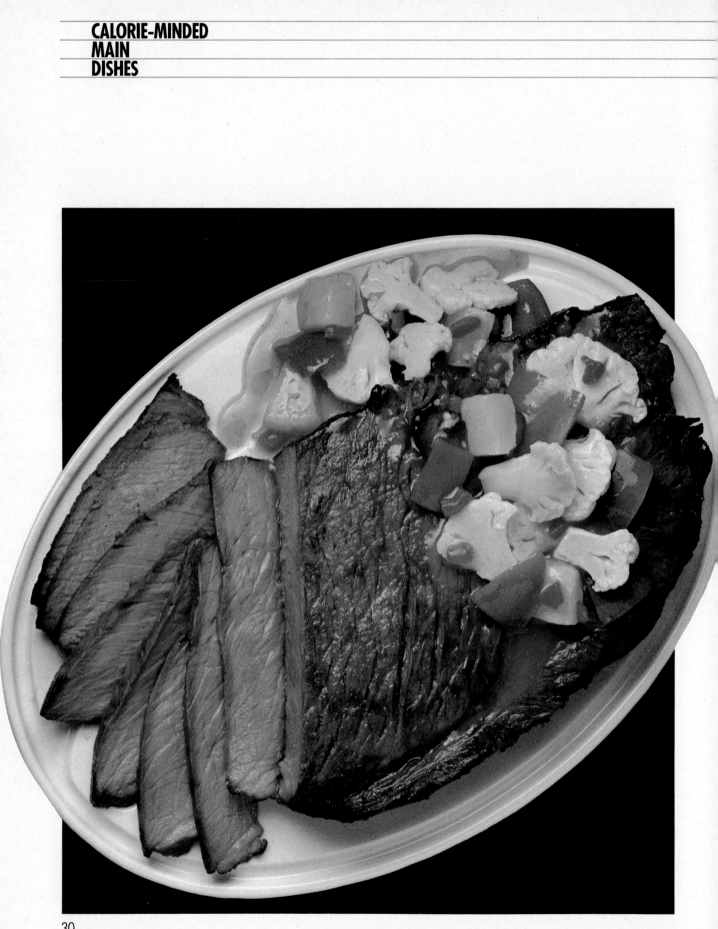

170 VEAL CHOP SUEY

Add 112 calories per ½ cup of hot cooked long grain rice or 110 calories per ½-cup serving of chow mein noodles—

Nonstick vegetable spray coating
1 pound boneless veal, cut into ¾-inch cubes
1½ cups water
3 tablespoons soy sauce
1 teaspoon instant chicken bouillon granules
1½ cups bias-sliced celery (about 5½ ounces)
1 medium onion, cut into wedges
1 16-ounce can bean sprouts, drained
1 cup frozen peas
1 cup sliced fresh mushrooms
2 tablespoons cold water
4 teaspoons cornstarch
Hot cooked rice or heated chow mein noodles (optional)

Spray the bottom of a large skillet with the nonstick vegetable spray coating. In the prepared skillet brown the veal cubes. Add the 1½ cups water, the soy sauce, and instant chicken bouillon granules. Cover and simmer about 25 minutes or till meat is tender.

Add the celery and onion. Cook for 5 minutes, stirring occasionally. Add the bean sprouts, frozen peas, and sliced mushrooms. Combine the 2 tablespoons cold water and the cornstarch; stir into meat mixture. Cook and stir till mixture is thickened and bubbly. Cook and stir 2 minutes more or till vegetables are crisp-tender. If desired, serve with hot cooked rice or heated chow mein noodles. Makes 6 servings.

◄ **Thinly slice the round steak across the grain when serving *Teriyaki Marinated Steak* with sweet-and-sour vegetables. Cover each portion of meat with some of the colorful vegetable mixture.**

180 TERIYAKI MARINATED STEAK

½ cup dry sherry
1 tablespoon soy sauce
1 tablespoon grated gingerroot or 1 teaspoon ground ginger
1 clove garlic, minced
1½ pounds boneless beef round steak, cut 1½ inches thick and trimmed of fat
1 cup sliced cauliflower flowerets
½ cup water
1 8-ounce can pineapple chunks (juice pack)
1 2-ounce jar sliced pimiento
1 tablespoon cornstarch
1 medium green pepper, cut into 1-inch squares
1 tablespoon vinegar
1 teaspoon paprika
½ teaspoon instant beef bouillon granules

For marinade, combine the sherry, soy sauce, gingerroot, and garlic. Pierce all surfaces of meat with a long-tined fork. Place meat in a plastic bag; set it in shallow dish. Add marinade to bag; close bag. Turn bag to coat all surfaces of meat. Refrigerate for 8 hours or overnight, turning bag several times to distribute marinade. Drain meat; reserve marinade. Pat meat dry with paper toweling. Place meat on rack of unheated broiler pan. Broil 4 inches from heat till meat reaches desired doneness, brushing occasionally with reserved marinade and turning once. Allow 14 to 16 minutes total for medium-rare.

Meanwhile, in medium saucepan cook cauliflower in the ½ cup water, covered, about 5 minutes or till just crisp-tender. Do not drain. Drain pineapple, reserving liquid. Set aside 2 teaspoons pimiento. In blender container puree the remaining pimiento; set aside. Combine cornstarch and pineapple liquid; add to cauliflower in saucepan. Add green pepper squares. Cook and stir till thickened and bubbly; cook and stir 2 minutes more. Stir in pineapple, the pureed pimiento, the 2 teaspoons reserved pimiento, vinegar, paprika, and bouillon granules; heat through. Slice meat across grain into thin slices. Top with vegetable mixture. Makes 6 servings.

184 VEAL PATTIES PARMESAN

1	beaten egg
1/3	cup soft bread crumbs (1/2 slice bread)
3	tablespoons grated Parmesan cheese
1	tablespoon finely chopped onion
1/4	teaspoon salt
1/8	teaspoon dried oregano, crushed
3/4	pound ground veal
1/3	cup tomato sauce
1/8	teaspoon dried oregano, crushed
1/8	teaspoon onion powder

In bowl combine egg, crumbs, Parmesan, onion, salt, 1/8 teaspoon oregano, and 1 tablespoon *water*. Add veal; mix well. Shape mixture into four 1/2-inch-thick patties. Place patties on rack of unheated broiler pan. Broil 3 inches from heat about 10 minutes or till done, turning once. Meanwhile, in small saucepan heat together tomato sauce, 1/8 teaspoon oregano, the onion powder, and 1 tablespoon *water*. To serve, spoon some sauce over each patty. Makes 4 servings.

166 ITALIAN VEAL STEAK

1	pound veal leg round steak, cut less than 1/2 inch thick
2	teaspoons cooking oil
1	7 1/2-ounce can tomatoes, cut up
1	tablespoon snipped parsley
2	teaspoons capers, drained
1/2	teaspoon Worcestershire sauce
1/4	teaspoon dried basil, crushed
	Dash salt
	Dash garlic powder

Cut veal into 4 pieces. Pound veal to 1/4- to 1/8-inch thickness (or have the butcher tenderize the steak). Brown meat quickly in hot cooking oil about 4 minutes, turning once. Remove veal and drain off fat. Combine *undrained* tomatoes, parsley, capers, Worcestershire sauce, basil, salt, and garlic powder in skillet. Simmer, covered, about 5 minutes. Return veal to skillet. Cover; simmer till heated through. To serve, spoon sauce over meat. Makes 4 servings.

138 DEVILED STEAK

1	pound beef sirloin steak, cut 1 inch thick and trimmed of fat
2	tablespoons dry sherry
1	tablespoon butter *or* margarine
1	teaspoon dry mustard
1	teaspoon Worcestershire sauce
	Dash pepper
1	tablespoon snipped parsley

Place the trimmed sirloin steak on rack of unheated broiler pan. Broil so surface of meat is 3 inches from heat. Broil steak to desired doneness; turn once (allow 8 to 10 minutes total time for rare, 12 to 14 minutes for medium, 18 to 20 minutes for well-done). In small saucepan combine sherry, butter or margarine, dry mustard, Worcestershire sauce, and pepper; heat till bubbly. Stir in parsley; spoon sauce over steak. Makes 4 servings.

143 OVEN-STYLE SWISS STEAK

1	pound boneless beef round steak, cut 1 inch thick and trimmed of fat
1/2	teaspoon salt
1/8	teaspoon pepper
1/2	medium onion, sliced
1	2-ounce can mushroom stems and pieces, drained
1/2	cup tomato sauce
1/4	teaspoon dried oregano, crushed

Cut meat into 4 portions; pound to 1/4-inch thickness. Sprinkle with the salt and pepper. Place meat in a 10x6x2-inch baking dish, overlapping slightly. Top with onion and mushrooms. Combine tomato sauce and oregano; pour sauce over all. Bake, covered, in a 350° oven for 1 1/4 hours. Uncover; bake about 15 minutes more. Baste occasionally. To serve, skim off any fat; spoon sauce over meat. Makes 4 servings.

160 TUNA-LETTUCE BUNDLES

2 large romaine leaves (1¾ ounces)
¼ cup finely chopped celery
3 tablespoons plain low-fat yogurt
2 tablespoons finely chopped onion
¼ teaspoon dried dillweed
1 3¼-ounce can tuna (water pack), drained

Remove heavy center veins from bottoms of romaine leaves. Combine the celery, yogurt, onion, and dillweed. Flake tuna and gently fold into yogurt mixture. Divide mixture between the romaine leaves. Fold all sides, envelope style. Place on plate. Cover with moistened paper toweling and refrigerate at least 30 minutes. Makes 1 serving.

156 SEAFOOD ROLLS

Pictured on pages 24 and 25 and on cover—

1 pound fresh *or* frozen flounder *or* sole fillets
½ cup shredded Swiss cheese (2 ounces)
1 2½-ounce jar sliced mushrooms, drained
¼ cup plain low-fat yogurt
1 tablespoon snipped chives
1 tablespoon chopped pimiento
½ teaspoon salt
⅛ teaspoon pepper
Nonstick vegetable spray coating
2 tablespoons fine dry bread crumbs
¼ teaspoon paprika
1 tablespoon plain low-fat yogurt

Thaw fish, if frozen. Cut fish into four portions, overlapping small pieces as necessary to make four rectangles. In a bowl combine the shredded cheese, drained mushrooms, the ¼ cup yogurt, the chives, pimiento, salt, and pepper. Spread mixture on fish. Roll up fillets around filling and place, seam side down, in a 10x6x2-inch baking dish that has been sprayed with nonstick vegetable spray coating.

Combine the bread crumbs and paprika. Brush fish with the 1 tablespoon yogurt and sprinkle with the bread crumb mixture. Bake in a 350° oven for 20 to 30 minutes or till the fish flakes easily when tested with a fork. Makes 4 servings.

143 ITALIAN SAUCED FISH

1 16-ounce package frozen flounder fillets
½ cup meatless spaghetti sauce
1 tablespoon chopped onion
1 tablespoon chopped green pepper
½ cup shredded mozzarella cheese (2 ounces)

Unwrap fish; let stand at room temperature about 20 minutes. Cut block of fish crosswise into 4 portions. Place fish in a 10x6x2-inch baking dish. Sprinkle lightly with salt. Combine the spaghetti sauce, onion, and green pepper; pour over fillets. Bake, uncovered, in a 450° oven about 20 minutes or till fish flakes easily when tested with a fork. Sprinkle with cheese; return to oven for about 3 minutes or till cheese melts. Serves 4.

194 ORANGE HALIBUT STEAKS

1 pound frozen halibut steaks
½ cup water
2 tablespoons frozen orange juice concentrate, thawed
1 tablespoon snipped parsley
1 tablespoon lemon juice
½ teaspoon dried dillweed
¼ teaspoon salt
Nonstick vegetable spray coating
4 thin orange slices, quartered *or* twisted (optional)

Thaw fish. Cut fish into 4 portions; place fish in shallow pan. Combine water, orange juice concentrate, parsley, lemon juice, dillweed, and salt; pour over fish. Marinate 30 minutes; turn once. Remove fish; reserve marinade. Spray broiler rack with nonstick vegetable spray coating. Place fish on rack of unheated broiler pan. Broil 4 inches from heat for 6 minutes. Turn; broil for 5 to 6 minutes or till fish flakes easily. Baste with reserved marinade. To serve, spoon any remaining marinade over fillets. Garnish with orange slices if desired. Makes 4 servings.

134 SHRIMP-STUFFED TOMATOES

   4 **large tomatoes**
   ¼ **cup chopped onion**
   ¼ **cup chopped celery**
   2 **tablespoons chopped green pepper**
   ¼ **teaspoon dried basil, crushed, *or* dillweed**
   2 **4½-ounce cans shrimp, rinsed, drained, and chopped (2 cups)**
   ½ **cup croutons**

Cut tops off tomatoes; scoop out pulp. Chop tops and pulp; drain well. In saucepan combine tomato pulp, onion, celery, green pepper, herb, and dash *pepper*. Simmer, covered, for 10 to 15 minutes or till vegetables are tender. Stir in shrimp and croutons. Pile shrimp mixture into tomato shells. Place in a 10x6x2-inch baking dish. Bake in a 375° oven for 20 to 25 minutes. Serves 4.

161 SALMON-STUFFED TOMATOES

   1 **15½-ounce can pink salmon, drained**
   1 **cup low-fat cottage cheese, drained**
   ½ **cup chopped celery**
   ¼ **cup Garden Yogurt Dressing**
   2 **tablespoons chopped green pepper**
   6 **medium tomatoes, chilled**
   6 **lettuce leaves**
   6 **lemon wedges**

In bowl flake salmon, removing bones and skin. Add cottage cheese, celery, dressing, green pepper, and dash *pepper*. Mix well; cover and chill. With stem end down, cut each tomato into 6 wedges, cutting to *but not through,* base of tomato. Spread wedges apart slightly. Sprinkle with ¼ teaspoon *salt*. Spoon about ⅓ cup mixture into *each* tomato. Serve tomatoes on lettuce-lined plates. Serve with lemon. Makes 6 servings.

Garden Yogurt Dressing: Mix ½ cup plain low-fat *yogurt*; ¼ cup peeled, seeded, and finely chopped *tomato*; 2 tablespoons finely chopped *green pepper*; 1 tablespoon chopped *green onion*; ⅛ teaspoon *salt*; ⅛ teaspoon *pepper*; and dash bottled *hot pepper sauce*. Cover; chill. Makes about ¾ cup. (7 calories/tablespoon).

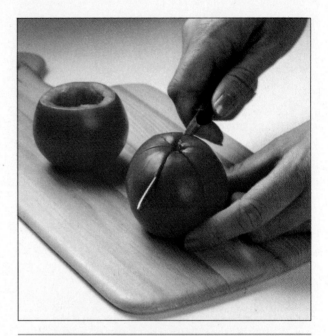

▲ MAKING TOMATO SHELLS

There are two ways you can prepare tomato shells for stuffing. One is to make petal cups by cutting a tomato into wedge-shaped pieces. To do this, place tomato, stem end down, on a cutting surface. Use a sharp knife to cut it into 4 to 6 wedges, cutting to *but not through,* the base of the tomato as shown. Spread the wedges apart slightly. Cover and chill the prepared tomato until you are ready to fill it.

Another way to prepare the shells is to cut a small slice from top of the tomato. Remove the core and use a spoon to scoop out the seeds, leaving a ½-inch-thick shell. If desired, you can add a sawtooth or scalloped edge to the shells using a sharp knife. Invert the tomatoes to drain. Cover and chill the tomatoes until you are ready to use them.

181 SCALLOP TOSS

- 1 **12-ounce package frozen scallops, thawed**
- 1 **clove garlic, halved**
- 2 **cups torn lettuce**
- 2 **cups torn romaine**
- 2 **cups torn spinach**
- 3 **hard-cooked eggs, sliced**
- ½ **cup sliced celery**
- 4 **ounces mozzarella cheese, cut into thin strips**
- ⅓ **cup Diet Russian Dressing (see recipe, page 62)**

Halve large scallops. In a saucepan cook scallops over low heat in a small amount of lightly salted boiling water for 2 to 3 minutes. Drain; cover and chill.

Rub a salad bowl with the garlic halves; discard garlic. In the salad bowl arrange lettuce, romaine, spinach, hard-cooked egg slices, celery, mozzarella cheese strips, and chilled scallops. Pour the Diet Russian Dressing over and toss to coat. Makes 6 servings.

196 MANDARIN-TUNA-RICE TOSS

You'll be surprised at the generous servings—

- 1¾ **cups cold cooked rice**
- 1 **9¼-ounce can tuna (water pack), drained and flaked**
- 1 **cup sliced celery**
- ½ **of an 11-ounce can mandarin orange sections, drained (½ cup)**
- ¼ **cup chopped green pepper**
- 2 **tablespoons sliced green onion**
- ¾ **cup plain low-fat yogurt**
- ¼ **teaspoon onion powder**
- 4 **lettuce leaves**

In a bowl combine the cooked rice, flaked tuna, sliced celery, mandarin oranges, green pepper, and green onion. Chill. In a small bowl stir together the yogurt and onion powder. Pour over the tuna mixture and toss lightly. Spoon salad onto lettuce leaves on individual plates. Serve immediately. Makes 4 servings.

137 EASY HERBED FISH

- 1 **pound fresh** or **frozen flounder** or **sole fillets**
  Freshly ground pepper
- 2 **tablespoons mayonnaise** or **salad dressing**
- 1½ **teaspoons finely chopped fresh tarragon leaves** or **½ teaspoon dried tarragon, crushed**
- ½ **teaspoon Dijon-style mustard**
  Paprika
- 4 **orange wedges**

Thaw fish, if frozen. Divide fish into 4 portions. Place fish on greased rack of unheated broiler pan, tucking under any thin edges. Sprinkle fish with freshly ground pepper. In bowl combine mayonnaise or salad dressing, tarragon, and mustard. Spread evenly over the fish. Broil 4 inches from heat for 5 to 7 minutes or till fish flakes easily when tested with a fork. Sprinkle top with paprika. Serve with orange wedges. Serves 4.

93 VEGETABLE-FISH BAKE

- 1 **16-ounce package frozen flounder** or **cod fillets**
  Nonstick vegetable spray coating
- 3 **tablespoons lemon juice**
- ½ **teaspoon paprika**
- ⅛ **teaspoon salt**
- 1 **cup sliced fresh mushrooms**
- 1 **small tomato, peeled and chopped**
- ¼ **cup chopped green pepper**
- 1 **tablespoon snipped parsley**
  Lemon wedges (optional)

Thaw fish fillets and cut into 4 portions. Spray a 10x6x2-inch baking dish with nonstick vegetable spray coating. Place fish pieces in baking dish; drizzle with the lemon juice and sprinkle with the paprika and salt. Combine the mushrooms, tomato, green pepper, and parsley. Sprinkle atop fish. Bake, covered, in a 350° oven about 25 minutes or till fish flakes easily when tested with a fork. Serve with lemon wedges if desired. Serves 4.

208 HAM AND CHEESE MEDLEY

1   8-ounce can pineapple chunks (juice pack), drained
5   ounces fully cooked ham, trimmed of fat and cubed (1 cup)
1   cup halved and seeded green grapes (6 ounces)
2   ounces Swiss cheese, cut into thin strips
¾   cup dry cottage cheese
½   cup skim milk
¼   teaspoon salt
1½ teaspoons snipped chives
4   cups torn lettuce

In a large bowl combine the pineapple chunks, ham, grapes, and Swiss cheese. Cover and chill. For dressing, in blender container combine dry cottage cheese, skim milk, and salt. Cover and blend about 20 seconds or till smooth. Stir in the snipped chives. Cover and chill.

To serve, toss lettuce with the ham and fruit mixture. Serve the salad mixture in individual salad bowls and pass the cottage cheese dressing. Makes 4 servings.

260 HAM-AND-EGGERS

4   slices whole wheat bread
4   ¾-ounce slices boiled ham (3 ounces total)
¼   cup plain low-fat yogurt
1   teaspoon prepared mustard
3   hard-cooked eggs, chopped
2   tablespoons finely chopped celery
1   tablespoon finely chopped green onion
4   slices mozzarella cheese (4 ounces)

Toast slices of bread. Place one ham slice atop each toast slice. In a bowl combine the yogurt and mustard. Stir in eggs, celery, and green onion. Divide the mixture among the four sandwiches and spread atop the ham. Place on rack of unheated broiler pan and broil 4 inches from heat for 3 to 4 minutes. Remove from broiler; top each with a slice of cheese. Return to broiler and broil about 1 minute or till cheese melts. Serves 4.

258 TANGERINE BROILED HAM

1   pound fully cooked ham, trimmed of fat and cut into 4 portions
¼   cup frozen tangerine juice concentrate, thawed
1½ teaspoons prepared mustard
¼   teaspoon ground ginger
1   medium orange *or* tangerine, thinly sliced

Place ham pieces in shallow baking dish. Combine the tangerine juice concentrate, mustard, ginger, and 2 tablespoons *water*. Pour over ham. Marinate 30 minutes, turning ham pieces once. Remove ham from marinade and place on rack of unheated broiler pan. Broil ham about 3 inches from heat for 2 to 3 minutes per side; brush often with reserved marinade. Add the orange or tangerine slices to broiler pan the last few minutes of broiling. (*Or,* grill ham over *hot* coals about 2 minutes on each side or till heated through. Brush often with reserved marinade. Heat orange slices on grill the last minute of cooking.) Serve the orange slices atop ham pieces. Serves 4.

279 HAM AND BULGUR SKILLET

⅓   cup sliced green onion
2   cloves garlic, minced
1   tablespoon butter *or* margarine
3   cups water
1   teaspoon instant beef bouillon granules
1   teaspoon dried oregano, crushed
    Dash pepper
1   cup bulgur wheat
6   ounces fully cooked ham, trimmed of fat and cut into bite-size pieces
1   9-ounce package frozen Italian green beans

Cook onion and garlic in butter till tender. Stir in water, bouillon granules, oregano, and pepper; bring to boiling. Stir in bulgur; reduce heat. Cover; simmer 15 minutes. Stir in ham and beans. Cover; simmer 10 minutes more. Makes 4 servings.

247 PORK CHOPS ITALIANO

4 pork loin chops, cut ¾ inch thick and
    trimmed of fat (about 1¾ pounds total)
2 teaspoons cooking oil
1 small onion, sliced
½ teaspoon dried marjoram, crushed
⅛ teaspoon garlic powder
⅛ teaspoon pepper
½ cup water

In a large skillet brown the pork chops in hot cooking oil. Remove chops from pan. In same skillet cook the sliced onion till tender; push to one side. Arrange pork chops in skillet; spoon onions atop. Combine marjoram, garlic powder, and pepper; sprinkle over meat. Add the water. Simmer, covered, over low heat for 35 to 40 minutes or till tender. Spoon juices over meat to serve. Makes 4 servings.

224 PINEAPPLE PORK CHOPS

6 pork loin rib chops, cut ½ inch thick and
    trimmed of fat (2 pounds total)
1 tablespoon cooking oil
½ teaspoon salt
⅛ teaspoon pepper
1 20-ounce can pineapple chunks (juice pack)
½ of a medium onion, thinly sliced
¼ teaspoon ground ginger
1 tablespoon cold water
1 teaspoon cornstarch

In a skillet brown the chops on both sides in hot cooking oil. Drain off fat. Season chops with the salt and pepper. Drain the pineapple chunks, reserving *½ cup* of the liquid. Arrange onion slices over chops. Top with reserved pineapple juice and pineapple chunks and sprinkle with the ginger. Cover and simmer about 40 minutes or till chops are tender. Remove chops from the skillet. Combine cold water and cornstarch. Stir into mixture in skillet. Cook and stir till mixture is thickened and bubbly. Cook and stir 2 minutes more. Serve pineapple sauce over chops. Serves 6.

TRIMMING MEAT

Cut calories by carefully trimming as much of the fat as possible from meats and poultry before cooking. Use a sharp knife. Be sure to skim off any excess fat that cooks out of the meat before serving sauce or gravy.

215 HAM AND VEGETABLE KABOBS

3 medium carrots, cut into 1-inch chunks
1 10-ounce package frozen brussels sprouts
¼ cup white wine vinegar
2 tablespoons cooking oil
1 tablespoon water
1 teaspoon Worcestershire sauce
½ teaspoon dried basil, crushed
¼ teaspoon dried rosemary, crushed
    Dash bottled hot pepper sauce
1 pound fully cooked ham, trimmed of fat
    and cut into 1-inch cubes

In a saucepan cook carrots, covered, in boiling water 12 to 15 minutes; drain. Cook brussels sprouts, covered, in boiling water 5 to 7 minutes; drain. In bowl combine the wine vinegar, oil, water, Worcestershire sauce, basil, rosemary, and hot pepper sauce. Stir in the carrots, brussels sprouts, and ham cubes. Cover and refrigerate several hours, stirring often.

Drain meat and vegetables, reserving marinade. Thread meat and vegetables alternately on 6 skewers. Place skewers on rack of unheated broiler pan. Broil 4 to 5 inches from heat for 5 minutes; brush with reserved marinade. Turn kabobs; brush with more marinade. Broil about 5 minutes more. Brush with marinade before serving. Makes 6 servings.

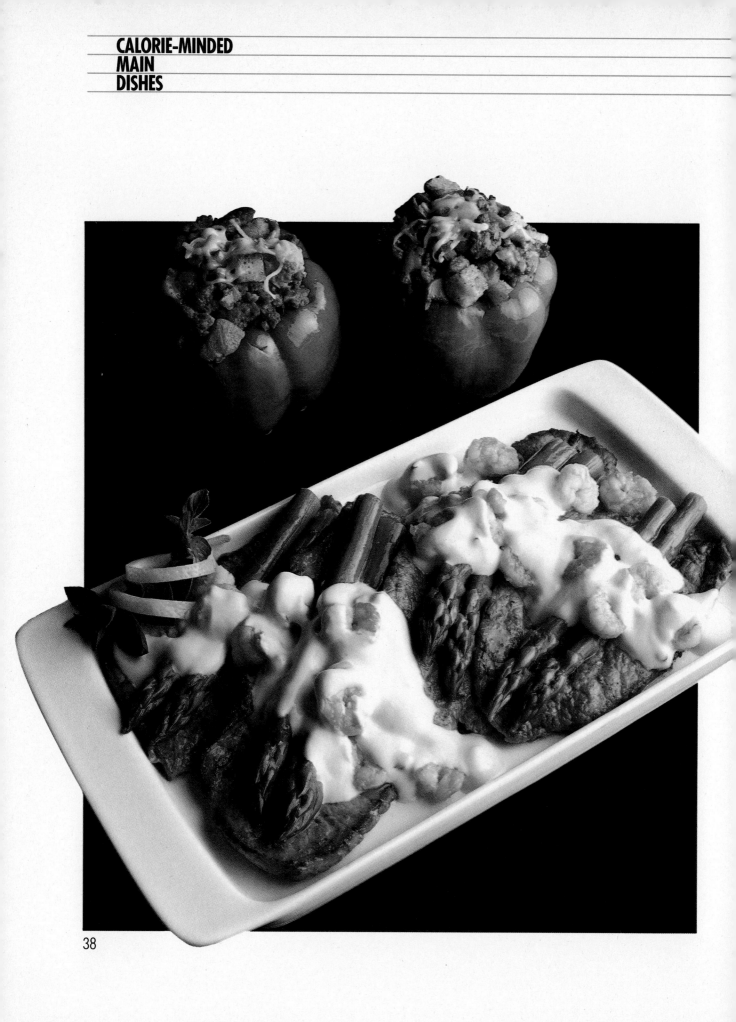

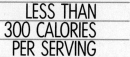
253 ELEGANT VEAL

- 1 pound veal leg round steak
- 1 tablespoon lemon juice
- ½ teaspoon salt
- ⅛ teaspoon pepper
- 1 tablespoon butter *or* margarine
- 1 4½-ounce can shrimp, drained
- 1 10-ounce package frozen asparagus spears
- ¼ cup dairy sour cream
- ¼ cup plain low-fat yogurt
- 1 teaspoon snipped chives
- 1 teaspoon lemon juice
- ½ teaspoon prepared mustard
- ¼ teaspoon dried tarragon, crushed

Cut veal into 4 pieces and pound with meat mallet to ¼-inch thickness. Sprinkle meat with the 1 tablespoon lemon juice, the salt, and pepper. In a large skillet heat butter or margarine till melted. Quickly cook veal two pieces at a time about 3 minutes or till browned. Turn and brown second side about 3 minutes. Remove meat from skillet and keep warm.

In a saucepan heat shrimp in 2 tablespoons *water*; drain. Cook asparagus according to package directions; drain. In small saucepan combine sour cream, yogurt, chives, the 1 teaspoon lemon juice, mustard, and tarragon. Cook and stir over very low heat till heated through; *do not boil*.

To serve, place veal on platter. Top each piece of meat with one-fourth of the cooked and drained asparagus spears and one-fourth of the drained shrimp. Divide the sour cream sauce over each serving. Makes 4 servings.

◄ *Elegant Veal*, topped with shrimp and asparagus spears, is fancy enough to serve guests. *Stuffed Peppers*, on the other hand, is an ideal ground meat dish to prepare for the family.

250 STUFFED PEPPERS

- 4 large green peppers
- ½ pound lean ground beef
- ¼ cup chopped onion
- 2 small tomatoes, peeled, seeded, and coarsely chopped (1 cup)
- ¾ cup herb-seasoned stuffing croutons
- ¾ cup shredded mozzarella cheese (3 ounces)
- 1 2-ounce can chopped mushrooms, drained
- ½ teaspoon Worcestershire sauce
- ¼ teaspoon garlic salt

Cut tops from green peppers; discard seeds and membranes. Chop tops to make ½ cup. Cook green pepper cups, uncovered, in boiling water for 5 minutes; invert to drain well. Sprinkle insides of peppers lightly with ⅛ teaspoon *salt*. In skillet cook the beef, the onion, and chopped green pepper tops till meat is browned and onion is tender; drain off fat. Stir in the chopped tomato, croutons, *½ cup* of the shredded cheese, the drained mushrooms, Worcestershire sauce, and the garlic salt. Spoon mixture into peppers. Place peppers in a 10x6x2-inch baking dish. Bake, covered, in a 350° oven 25 minutes. Uncover; sprinkle with remaining ¼ cup mozzarella cheese. Bake about 5 minutes more. Makes 4 servings.

253 BASIC MEAT LOAF

- 1 teaspoon instant beef bouillon granules
- 1 beaten egg
- 1½ cups soft bread crumbs
- ¼ cup chopped onion
- ½ teaspoon ground sage
- ¼ teaspoon salt
- 1 pound lean ground beef
- 3 tablespoons chili sauce

Dissolve bouillon granules in ¼ cup hot *water*. Combine with egg, crumbs, onion, sage, salt, and dash *pepper*. Add beef; mix well. Shape into a loaf about 6x4 inches; place in a 10x6x2-inch baking dish. Bake in a 350° oven for 45 minutes. Drain off fat. Spread chili sauce over loaf. Bake 10 to 15 minutes more. Makes 5 servings.

294 GARDEN SANDWICH

Pictured on page 16—

1½ ounces thinly sliced cooked beef
    rump roast, trimmed of fat
½ ounce sliced mozzarella cheese
2 lettuce leaves
1 small tomato, sliced
¼ small cucumber, sliced
1 frankfurter bun, split
1 tablespoon low-calorie Italian salad
    dressing (no more than 8 calories per
    tablespoon)

Place beef, cheese, lettuce, tomato, and cucumber in bun. Drizzle dressing between layers. For brown bag lunch, place meat and cheese in bun; wrap. Pack lettuce in one container and tomato, cucumber, and dressing in another. Keep all cold. Assemble when ready to eat. Serves 1.

219 LOW-CAL MOUSSAKA

¾ pound lean ground lamb
¼ cup chopped onion
2 cups peeled and coarsely chopped eggplant
1 7½-ounce can tomatoes, cut up
1 2-ounce can chopped mushrooms, drained
2 tablespoons snipped parsley
½ teaspoon dried oregano, crushed
¼ teaspoon dried rosemary, crushed
¼ teaspoon ground cinnamon
1 egg
3 ounces Neufchâtel cheese, cut up
½ cup plain low-fat yogurt

Cook lamb and onion till meat is browned. Drain off fat thoroughly. Stir in eggplant, *undrained* tomatoes, mushrooms, parsley, oregano, rosemary, ⅛ *teaspoon* of the cinnamon, and ½ teaspoon *salt*. Cook, uncovered, 15 minutes, stirring occasionally. Turn into a 10x6x2-inch baking dish. Place egg, cheese, yogurt, remaining cinnamon, and ⅛ teaspoon *salt* in blender container. Cover; blend till smooth. Pour atop meat. Bake in a 350° oven 15 to 20 minutes or till yogurt mixture is set. Garnish with parsley if desired. Serves 4.

273 DIET TACO BURGERS

Pictured on pages 10 and 11—

1 beaten egg
1 7½-ounce can tomatoes, cut up
3 tablespoons wheat germ
2 tablespoons finely chopped onion
1 tablespoon chopped canned green chili
    peppers
½ teaspoon salt
¾ pound lean ground beef
1 tablespoon chopped canned green
    chili peppers
2 teaspoons cornstarch
¼ teaspoon ground cumin
    Few dashes bottled hot pepper sauce
1 small head lettuce, coarsely
    shredded
¼ cup shredded Monterey Jack
    cheese (1 ounce)

In bowl combine egg, *2 tablespoons* of the *undrained* tomatoes, wheat germ, onion, 1 tablespoon canned green chili peppers, and salt. Add ground beef and mix well. Shape meat mixture into four ½-inch-thick patties. Place patties on rack of unheated broiler pan. Broil 3 inches from heat, turning meat patties once. Allow about 10 minutes total broiling time for medium doneness. (Or, grill patties over *medium* coals, turning once. Allow 12 to 15 minutes total grilling time for medium doneness.)

Meanwhile, in a saucepan stir together remaining *undrained* tomatoes, 1 tablespoon canned green chili peppers, cornstarch, cumin, and hot pepper sauce. Cook and stir till mixture is thickened and bubbly. Cook and stir 2 minutes more. To serve, place a beef patty on a bed of shredded lettuce; top with some of the tomato mixture and sprinkle each serving with some of the Monterey Jack cheese. Makes 4 servings.

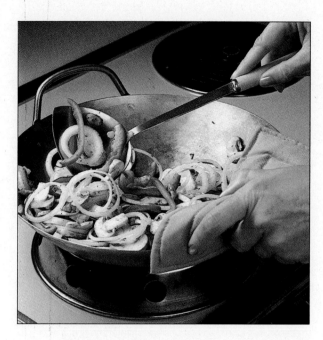

287 STUFFED CABBAGE ROLLS FOR TWO

1 beaten egg
2 tablespoons wheat germ
1 teaspoon minced dried onion
¼ teaspoon salt
¼ teaspoon caraway seed
⅓ pound lean ground beef
⅓ cup cold cooked rice
4 medium cabbage leaves (6 ounces)
½ cup tomato sauce
½ teaspoon dried basil, crushed

In a bowl combine the egg, wheat germ, onion, salt, caraway seed, and dash *pepper*; mix well. Add the beef and rice; mix well. Remove the center vein of cabbage leaves, keeping each leaf in one piece. Immerse leaves in boiling water about 3 minutes or till limp; drain. Place about *¼ cup* of the mixture on each leaf; fold in the sides. Starting at unfolded edge, roll up each leaf, making sure folded sides are included in roll. Arrange in a 10x6x2-inch baking dish. Stir together the tomato sauce and basil. Pour over cabbage rolls. Bake, uncovered, in a 350° oven for 30 to 35 minutes. Skim any fat from sauce. Makes 2 servings.

◄ **STIR-FRY COOKING**
Equipment for this popular method of cooking includes a wok or large skillet and a long-handled spoon or wide spatula. Oil is often heated in the wok before food is added. Use the utensil to lift and turn the food with a folding motion as shown. Cook food quickly when stir-frying to achieve the desired crisp-tender texture of certain vegetables. The frequent lifting and turning results in even cooking.

243 STIR-FRIED GAZPACHO SALAD

Pictured on pages 24 and 25—

1 pound beef round steak, trimmed of fat
2 tablespoons cooking oil
1 clove garlic, minced
8 ounces fresh mushrooms, sliced (3 cups)
1 small cucumber, seeded and coarsely chopped
1 medium green pepper, cut into strips
1 medium onion, sliced and separated into rings
1 teaspoon Italian seasoning
1 teaspoon seasoned salt
⅛ teaspoon ground red pepper
1 large tomato, cut into wedges
8 ounces fresh spinach leaves (6 cups)

Partially freeze beef; slice thinly across the grain into bite-size strips. In wok or large skillet cook *half* of the beef in hot oil till browned on all sides. Remove from pan. Repeat with remaining beef and the garlic; remove from pan. Add mushrooms, cucumber, green pepper, onion, Italian seasoning, seasoned salt, and red pepper to wok. Stir-fry 3 minutes or till vegetables are crisp-tender. Add meat and tomato to wok; cook 1 to 2 minutes or till heated through. Remove meat-vegetable mixture to serving bowl; keep warm. Add spinach leaves to wok; cover and cook for 1 minute or till slightly wilted. To serve, arrange wilted spinach leaves on four plates or bowls; spoon meat-vegetable mixture atop. Serves 4.

41

► **BROILING FOR LEAN EATING**
Broiling allows the fat to drip away from the food as it cooks. To broil, place foods to be cooked on the rack of an unheated broiler pan. Improvise with a wire rack and shallow baking pan if you don't have a broiler pan. Use a ruler to measure the distance from the top of the food to the heat source (as shown). Cook the food according to recipe directions.

BELL PEPPERS
238 WITH EGGPLANT STUFFING

4   medium green peppers
3   cups peeled and cubed eggplant (8 ounces)
⅓   cup chopped onion
1   clove garlic, minced
½   teaspoon salt
⅛   teaspoon ground red pepper
¾   pound lean ground beef, cooked and
      drained thoroughly
1   beaten egg
2   tablespoons skim milk
    Nonstick vegetable spray coating
3   tablespoons soft bread crumbs
2   tablespoons snipped parsley

Cut tops from green peppers; discard seeds and membranes and reserve tops from peppers. Cook the whole green peppers, uncovered, in boiling water for 5 minutes; invert to drain well.

Chop tops of green peppers. In saucepan combine chopped pepper, eggplant, onion, garlic, salt, and red pepper. Cook, covered, about 5 minutes or till tender. Drain. Remove from heat. Add drained ground beef. Mix well. Combine egg and milk. Add *half* the beef mixture to egg and milk; return all to saucepan. Mix well. Fill peppers with eggplant mixture. Arrange peppers in an 8x8x2-inch baking dish that has been sprayed with nonstick vegetable spray coating. Bake stuffed peppers in a 350° oven for 20 minutes. Combine bread crumbs and parsley; sprinkle atop stuffed peppers. Bake about 5 minutes or till bread crumbs are lightly toasted. Serves 4.

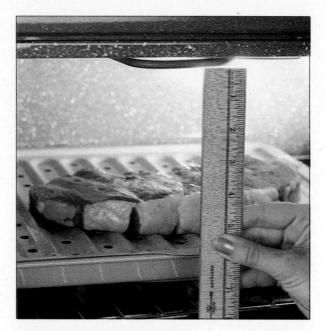

269 REUBEN MEAT LOAF

1   beaten egg
1   cup soft rye bread crumbs
½   cup chopped onion
¼   cup reduced-calorie Russian salad dressing
      (no more than 25 calories per tablespoon)
1   tablespoon Worcestershire sauce
1   teaspoon salt
¼   teaspoon pepper
1½ pounds lean ground beef
1   8-ounce can sauerkraut, drained and finely
      snipped
1   cup shredded Swiss cheese (4 ounces)

In a bowl combine egg, bread crumbs, onion, salad dressing, Worcestershire sauce, salt, and pepper. Add ground beef and mix well. On waxed paper pat mixture into a 12x8-inch rectangle. Top with the sauerkraut and ¾ *cup* of the cheese. Using waxed paper to lift rectangle, roll up meat jelly-roll style, beginning with short side. Press ends to seal. Place roll, seam side down, in a 13x9x2-inch baking pan. Bake in a 350° oven for 50 minutes. Sprinkle remaining cheese atop. Bake about 3 minutes more. Makes 8 servings.

212 STUFFED STEAKS

1¼ **pounds boneless beef round steak, cut**
 ½ inch thick and trimmed of fat
¼ **teaspoon salt**
⅛ **teaspoon pepper**
⅓ **cup low-calorie French salad dressing**
 (no more than 15 calories per tablespoon)
⅔ **cup shredded carrot**
½ **cup finely chopped onion**
½ **cup finely chopped green pepper**
½ **cup finely chopped celery**
½ **cup water**
¼ **teaspoon salt**
½ **cup beef broth**
1 **tablespoon cornstarch**
1 **tablespoon cold water**
¼ **teaspoon Kitchen Bouquet**

Cut meat into 4 rectangular portions. Pound meat to ¼-inch thickness. Sprinkle meat with ¼ teaspoon salt and the pepper. Brush with salad dressing. Place in shallow dish; marinate for 30 to 60 minutes at room temperature.

In saucepan combine carrot, onion, green pepper, celery, ½ cup water, and ¼ teaspoon salt. Simmer, covered, 7 to 8 minutes or till vegetables are crisp-tender. Drain.

Place about ¼ cup of the vegetable mixture on each piece of steak. Roll up jelly-roll style; secure with wooden picks. Place meat rolls in an 8-inch skillet; pour beef broth over meat. Simmer, covered, 35 to 40 minutes or till tender.

Transfer meat to serving platter; remove and discard wooden picks. Skim fat from broth; reserve 1 cup of the broth. Combine cornstarch, 1 tablespoon cold water, and the Kitchen Bouquet; stir into reserved broth. Cook and stir till thickened and bubbly; cook and stir 2 minutes more. Pour sauce over meat rolls. Makes 4 servings.

237 BROILED LIVER WITH MUSHROOMS

1 **cup sliced fresh mushrooms**
¼ **cup low-calorie French salad dressing**
 (no more than 15 calories per tablespoon)
¾ **pound calf liver, sliced ½ inch thick**
 Snipped parsley (optional)

Marinate mushrooms in dressing 30 minutes. Remove any hard portions or veins present in liver. Cut into 4 serving-size pieces. Drain mushrooms; reserve marinade. Brush both sides of liver with reserved marinade. Place liver on rack of unheated broiler pan. Broil 3 inches from heat for 3 minutes. Turn; top liver with drained mushrooms and broil for 3 to 4 minutes longer or till liver is done. Trim with parsley if desired. Serves 4.

229 LEMON-SAUCED VEAL MEATBALLS

1 **beaten egg**
3 **tablespoons skim milk**
1 **cup soft bread crumbs (about 1½ slices)**
2 **tablespoons chopped onion**
3 **tablespoons snipped parsley**
1 **pound ground veal**
1 **tablespoon cornstarch**
 Dash white pepper
1 **cup skim milk**
1 **hard-cooked egg, chopped**
½ **teaspoon finely shredded lemon peel**
2 **tablespoons lemon juice**

In bowl combine egg and 3 tablespoons skim milk. Stir in crumbs, onion, 2 tablespoons of the parsley, and ½ teaspoon salt. Add veal; mix well. Shape into 30 meatballs. Place in shallow baking pan. Bake, uncovered, in a 375° oven for 25 to 30 minutes or till done. In a saucepan combine cornstarch, pepper, and ¼ teaspoon salt. Stir 1 cup skim milk into cornstarch mixture till smooth. Cook and stir till thickened and bubbly; stir in hard-cooked egg, lemon peel, and lemon juice. Cook and stir 2 minutes more. Spoon meatballs into serving dish, leaving any fat in baking pan. Pour lemon sauce over meatballs. Sprinkle with remaining snipped parsley. Makes 5 servings.

43

275 CHICKEN-BEEF KABOBS

½ pound boneless beef, trimmed of fat
1 whole large chicken breast (about 1 pound), skinned, halved, and boned
1 cup plain low-fat yogurt
¼ cup chopped onion
¼ cup skim milk
1 clove garlic, minced
1 teaspoon ground coriander
½ teaspoon ground cumin
4 small onions
2 medium zucchini, cut into 1-inch slices

Cut beef into 1-inch cubes and chicken into 1-inch pieces. For marinade mix next 6 ingredients and ½ teaspoon *salt*. Stir in the meats. Cover and refrigerate several hours; stir occasionally. Cook small onions in boiling salted water 5 minutes; drain. Preheat broiler. Drain meats; reserve the marinade. Alternately thread beef, zucchini, and chicken on skewers. Broil 4 to 5 inches from heat 8 minutes. Brush with marinade. Turn kabobs; brush with marinade. Broil 8 minutes. Brush with marinade; place an onion on each skewer. Turn; broil 6 minutes. Brush with marinade. Serves 4.

238 PEPPER CHICKEN AND SPROUTS

1 whole small chicken breast (8 ounces), skinned, halved lengthwise, and boned
1 medium green pepper
1 slightly beaten egg white
1 teaspoon cornstarch
1 tablespoon cooking oil
½ medium onion, thinly sliced
2 cups fresh lentil *or* bean sprouts
1 medium tomato, cut into thin wedges

Cut chicken and pepper into ½-inch pieces. Mix egg white, cornstarch, 2 teaspoons *water*, and ¼ teaspoon *salt*. Add chicken; toss to coat. Preheat skillet over high heat. Add oil. Add chicken, green pepper, and onion; stir-fry in oil over high heat 3 to 4 minutes or till chicken is done. Add sprouts; stir-fry 1 minute. Add tomato; cover and heat 2 minutes. Sprinkle with pepper. Makes 2 servings.

244 CHICKEN AND APPLES

2 whole medium chicken breasts (about 1½ pounds total), skinned, halved lengthwise, and boned
¼ cup chopped onion
¼ cup shredded carrot
1 tablespoon cooking oil
1 tablespoon cornstarch
1 teaspoon instant chicken bouillon granules
¼ teaspoon ground cinnamon
1 5½-ounce can (⅔ cup) apple juice
1 tablespoon vinegar
2 small apples, cored and cut into rings
1 tablespoon snipped parsley

Cut chicken into ½-inch-wide strips. In medium skillet cook onion and carrot in hot oil till tender but not brown. Add chicken pieces; cook till chicken is no longer pink. In a small bowl combine the cornstarch, bouillon granules, and cinnamon. Stir in the apple juice and vinegar till thoroughly combined. Add to chicken mixture in skillet. Cook and stir till thickened and bubbly. Place apple rings atop chicken mixture; cover and cook over medium-low heat about 3 minutes or till apple rings are tender. Transfer apple rings to platter; top with chicken mixture. Sprinkle with the snipped parsley. Makes 4 servings.

HOLIDAY DIETING TIPS

Here are some suggestions to help you cut calories without missing out on the holiday feasting:

● Select the white breast meat of turkey or chicken and remove the skin. Trim all fat from a meat roast before eating.

● Skip the commercial eggnog and make a lighter version with skim milk and less sugar or an artificial sweetener.

● At appetizer time, select fresh vegetables with only a small portion of dip.

270 CHICKEN-SAUCED SPAGHETTI

½ cup chopped onion
1 medium carrot, thinly sliced (½ cup)
1 cup tomato juice
2 tablespoons snipped parsley
½ to 1 teaspoon chili powder
½ teaspoon sugar
½ teaspoon dried oregano, crushed
2 teaspoons cornstarch
1½ cups cubed cooked chicken *or* turkey
2 cups hot cooked spaghetti

In a 1½-quart saucepan cook onion and carrot in ½ cup *water,* covered, for 8 to 10 minutes or till tender. Stir in tomato juice, parsley, chili powder, sugar, oregano, ¼ teaspoon *salt,* and ⅛ teaspoon *pepper.* Bring to boiling; reduce heat. Cover; simmer 10 minutes. Combine cornstarch and 2 tablespoons *cold water;* stir into mixture in saucepan. Cook and stir till bubbly; cook and stir 2 minutes more. Stir in cooked chicken; heat through. Serve over spaghetti. Makes 3 servings.

221 ELEGANT CHICKEN BREASTS

Pictured on page 23—

3 whole large chicken breasts (about 3 pounds total), skinned and halved lengthwise
¾ cup unsweetened pineapple juice
1½ teaspoons sugar
¼ teaspoon dried tarragon, crushed
2 teaspoons cornstarch
Paprika

Place chicken in a 10-inch skillet. Combine pineapple juice, sugar, tarragon, and ½ teaspoon *salt.* Pour juice mixture over chicken. Cover and cook over low heat about 25 minutes or till chicken is done. Transfer chicken to platter; keep warm. Skim excess fat from mixture in skillet. Combine cornstarch and 1 tablespoon *cold water.* Stir into sauce in skillet. Cook and stir till thickened and bubbly; cook and stir 2 minutes longer. Drizzle sauce over chicken. Sprinkle with paprika. Trim with parsley if desired. Serves 6.

231 SPICY TOMATO CHICKEN FOR TWO

1 whole medium chicken breast (12 ounces), skinned and halved lengthwise
1 medium onion, cut into small wedges
1 clove garlic, minced
1 tablespoon butter *or* margarine
1½ teaspoons paprika
¼ teaspoon ground coriander
¼ teaspoon ground cumin
¼ teaspoon ground turmeric
⅛ teaspoon ground cinnamon
Few dashes bottled hot pepper sauce
2 tablespoons tomato paste

Bone chicken if desired. In a skillet cook onion and garlic in butter till onion is tender but not brown. Add paprika, coriander, cumin, turmeric, cinnamon, pepper sauce, and ¼ teaspoon *salt.* Stir in tomato paste and ½ cup *water.* Add chicken pieces, turning to coat. Cover and simmer about 35 minutes or till chicken is tender; stir occasionally. Skim off excess fat if necessary. Serve with hot cooked rice if desired. Serves 2.

219 CHICKEN AND PINEAPPLE CURRY

1 12-ounce can vegetable juice cocktail
1 small onion, cut into small wedges
1½ to 2 teaspoons curry powder
1 teaspoon instant chicken bouillon granules
½ teaspoon poultry seasoning
1 3-pound broiler-fryer chicken, cut up
1 tablespoon all-purpose flour
1 8-ounce can pineapple chunks (juice pack)

In a skillet combine ½ cup of the vegetable juice cocktail and ½ cup *water.* Add onion, curry, bouillon granules, poultry seasoning, and dash *pepper.* Remove skin and fat from chicken. Add chicken to skillet, turning to coat. Cover; simmer 35 to 40 minutes or till tender. Remove chicken; keep warm. Skim fat from mixture in skillet. Combine remaining vegetable cocktail and flour. Add to skillet. Cook and stir till bubbly. Cook and stir 1 minute more. Drain pineapple. Stir pineapple into sauce; heat. Pour sauce over chicken. Serves 6.

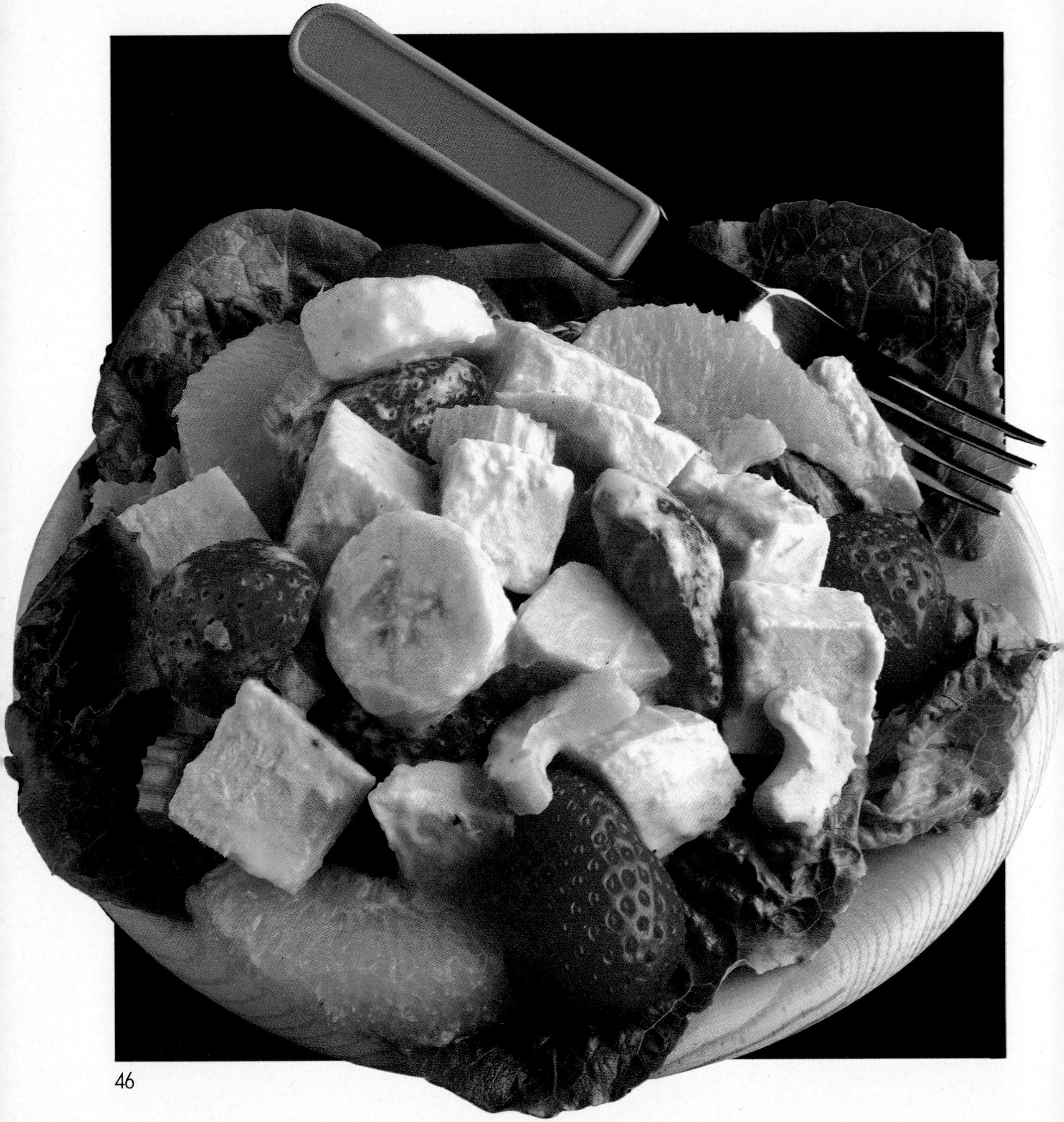

MINTED CHICKEN-
299 GRAPEFRUIT SALAD

Use the grapefruit shells as the serving containers for this main-dish salad for two—

2   medium grapefruit
2   ounces Neufchâtel cheese
1   tablespoon skim milk
2   teaspoons lemon juice
2   teaspoons honey
½   teaspoon dried mint, crushed
¾   cup cubed cooked chicken *or* turkey
     white meat (about 4 ounces)
1   small apple, cored and sliced
2   lettuce leaves (optional)
     Poppy seed

Cut slice from top third of each grapefruit. Remove fruit from grapefruit, leaving shells intact. (Use a grapefruit knife to remove the grapefruit meat.) Discard tops of grapefruit. Section grapefruit. If desired, cut top edge of each grapefruit shell in sawtooth fashion. Invert grapefruit shells on a paper-towel-lined tray. Chill.

In a small bowl beat together the Neufchâtel cheese, skim milk, lemon juice, and honey till smooth. Stir in the crushed dried mint; cover and chill the dressing.

In a bowl combine grapefruit sections, chicken or turkey, sliced apple, and mint dressing. If desired, line two individual serving plates with lettuce leaves. Place grapefruit shells on the serving plates. Spoon in the grapefruit mixture. Sprinkle the salads lightly with poppy seed. Serve at once. Makes 2 servings.

◄   **Next time you roast a turkey, cook enough to have extra to make *Turkey-Fruit Salad*. The fruits in this refreshing salad are strawberries, bananas, and oranges.**

CALORIE-CUTTING TIPS
● **Omit one slice of bread and serve sandwiches open-face. Use two extra-thin slices of bread for a two-slice sandwich.**
● **Instead of seasoning cooked vegetables with a pat of butter or margarine, try using a squeeze of lemon juice.**
● **Whenever possible, spray the pan with nonstick vegetable spray coating instead of using cooking oil or shortening to fry foods. Or, cook in a pan with a nonstick coating.**
● **Skim milk and reconstituted nonfat dry milk are good calorie cutters when cooking. Skim milk is good for drinking, too. One cup of whole milk has 159 calories, and one cup of skim milk has 88 calories.**

255 TURKEY-FRUIT SALAD

⅓   cup plain low-fat yogurt
1   tablespoon mayonnaise *or* salad dressing
1   tablespoon honey
½   teaspoon finely shredded orange peel
⅛   teaspoon salt
2   cups cubed cooked turkey *or* chicken
1   cup fresh strawberries, halved
1   small banana, cut into ½-inch slices
½   cup sliced celery
2   medium oranges
     Lettuce leaves

In a bowl stir together yogurt, mayonnaise or salad dressing, honey, orange peel, and the salt. Cover and chill. Combine turkey, strawberries, banana, and celery. Fold in the chilled yogurt mixture, mixing lightly to coat. Cover; chill up to 2 hours. Peel and section oranges. Arrange lettuce on individual serving plates. Arrange orange sections on each plate and mound turkey-fruit mixture in center. Makes 4 servings.

228 TUNA AND CHEESE WAFFLEWICHES

- 2 ounces Neufchâtel cheese, softened
- 1 to 2 tablespoons skim milk
- 1 3¼-ounce can tuna (water pack), drained and flaked
- 2 tablespoons chopped celery
- 1 teaspoon lemon juice
- ⅛ teaspoon dried dillweed
- 2 frozen waffles
- 2 cherry tomatoes, sliced into thirds

In a mixing bowl beat the cheese with enough of the milk to make creamy. Stir in the tuna, celery, lemon juice, and dillweed; mix well. Spread one-half of the mixture on each waffle. Place on baking sheet and bake in a 350° oven about 15 minutes or till heated through. Garnish with sliced cherry tomatoes. Makes 2 servings.

279 WINE-POACHED HALIBUT

- 4 fresh or frozen halibut steaks (about 1⅓ pounds total)
- ¾ cup dry white wine or water
- ½ cup water
- ½ cup sliced fresh mushrooms
- ¼ cup thinly sliced celery
- 1 clove garlic, minced
- ½ teaspoon dried mint, crushed
- ¼ teaspoon salt
- ⅛ teaspoon pepper
- Chopped pimiento
- Lemon wedges (optional)

Thaw fish if frozen. In a large skillet combine the ¾ cup wine, ½ cup water, mushrooms, celery, garlic, mint, salt, and pepper. Bring mixture to boiling; reduce heat. Simmer, covered, for 5 minutes. Add fish and spoon poaching liquid over fish. Simmer, covered, for 6 to 8 minutes or till fish flakes easily when tested with a fork. Transfer fish to platter; keep warm. Boil vegetable mixture, uncovered, for 3 to 6 minutes or till reduced to ½ to ⅔ cup. Spoon atop steaks. Sprinkle with the chopped pimiento. Garnish with lemon wedges if desired. Makes 4 servings.

264 TUNA-STUFFED POTATOES

- 2 baking potatoes (each about 5 inches long)
- 2 tablespoons skim milk
- ¼ teaspoon seasoned salt
- 1 3¼-ounce can tuna (water pack), drained
- ¼ cup shredded American cheese (1 ounce)
- 2 tablespoons chopped green pepper
- 1 tablespoon snipped chives
- Paprika

Scrub potatoes and bake in a 425° oven for 40 to 60 minutes or till done. Cut baked potatoes in half lengthwise. Reserving potato shells, scoop out the insides and mash with the skim milk and seasoned salt. Fold in the tuna, cheese, green pepper, and chives. Spoon mixture into potato shells. Sprinkle with paprika. Place on baking sheet. Bake, uncovered, in a 425° oven for 10 to 15 minutes or till heated through. Makes 2 servings.

244 COTTAGE CHEESE-TUNA SANDWICHES

- 1 6½-ounce can tuna (water pack), drained and flaked
- 1 cup low-fat cottage cheese
- ½ cup shredded Swiss cheese (2 ounces)
- 1 medium tomato, chopped
- ¼ cup chopped celery
- 2 tablespoons sliced green onion
- ⅓ cup plain low-fat yogurt
- ¼ teaspoon salt
- 4 slices thin-sliced whole wheat bread, toasted
- 1 cup fresh alfalfa sprouts

In a medium bowl combine the drained tuna, the cottage cheese, Swiss cheese, tomato, celery, and green onion. Stir together the yogurt and salt; fold into tuna mixture. Spread a generous ⅓ cup of the tuna mixture on each of the toast slices. Top each sandwich with ¼ cup of the alfalfa sprouts. Serve at once. Makes 4 servings.

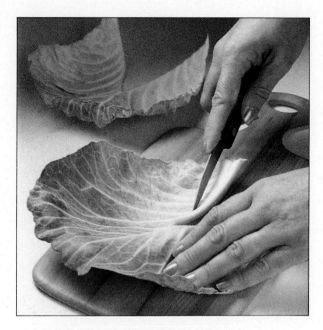

269 TUNA-MAC CASSEROLE

5   ounces elbow macaroni (1⅓ cups)
2   cups skim milk
2   tablespoons cornstarch
2   teaspoons minced dried onion
¾   teaspoon dried dillweed
½   teaspoon salt
    Dash pepper
1   cup cubed *or* shredded American cheese
    (4 ounces)
1   3¼-ounce can tuna (water pack), drained
    and flaked
1   medium tomato, sliced

Cook macaroni in boiling salted water according to package directions; drain. In saucepan combine skim milk, cornstarch, dried onion, dillweed, salt, and pepper. Cook and stir till thickened and bubbly. Add the cheese and stir till melted. Stir in the drained macaroni and the flaked tuna. Turn mixture into a 1½-quart casserole. Bake, uncovered, in a 350° oven for 20 minutes. Arrange tomato slices atop macaroni mixture. Continue baking 10 to 15 minutes more or till heated through. Makes 5 servings.

◀   **PREPARING CABBAGE FOR DOLMAS**
Remove the heavy center vein of cabbage leaves, keeping each leaf in one piece as shown. Cook cabbage leaves in boiling water till limp; drain. Add salmon mixture; fold in sides and tuck ends under. Place in baking dish, seam side down.

212 SALMON DOLMAS

1   beaten egg
¼   cup finely chopped onion
1   teaspoon Worcestershire sauce
¼   teaspoon salt
¼   teaspoon dried dillweed
1   15½-ounce can pink salmon, drained,
    flaked, and skin and bones removed
¾   cup hot cooked rice
6   large cabbage leaves
1   tablespoon butter *or* margarine
4   teaspoons all-purpose flour
¼   teaspoon salt
1   cup skim milk
½   cup shredded process Swiss cheese
1   tablespoon lemon juice
    Paprika

In bowl combine egg, onion, Worcestershire, ¼ teaspoon salt, dillweed, and dash *pepper*. Add salmon and rice; mix well. Remove heavy center vein of cabbage leaves, keeping each leaf in one piece (see tip above). Immerse cabbage leaves in boiling water about 3 minutes or till limp; drain. Place ⅓ *cup* of the salmon mixture on *each* leaf; fold in sides and tuck ends under. Place, seam side down, in a 10x6x2-inch baking dish. Cover with foil; bake in a 350° oven about 45 minutes.

For sauce, in a saucepan melt the butter or margarine; blend in flour, ¼ teaspoon salt, and dash *pepper*. Add milk; cook and stir till mixture is thickened and bubbly. Cook and stir 1 minute more. Remove sauce from heat; add the cheese and lemon juice. Stir till cheese melts. Serve cheese sauce over cabbage-salmon rolls. Sprinkle with paprika. Makes 6 servings.

257 SHRIMP THERMIDOR BAKE

¼ cup chopped onion
¼ cup chopped celery
1 11-ounce can condensed cheddar cheese soup
½ cup skim milk
2 tablespoons dry sherry
¾ pound fresh *or* frozen shelled shrimp, cooked
2 tablespoons snipped parsley
Dash bottled hot pepper sauce
¾ cup soft bread crumbs (1 slice)
1 tablespoon butter *or* margarine, melted
Dash paprika

In a covered saucepan cook onion and celery in a small amount of water for 5 minutes; drain. Stir condensed soup, milk, and sherry into vegetables in saucepan. Stir in shrimp, parsley, and hot pepper sauce. Spoon mixture into four individual baking shells. Toss together the bread crumbs, melted butter or margarine, and paprika. Sprinkle atop mixture in each shell. Bake in a 375° oven for 15 to 20 minutes. Makes 4 servings.

255 SHRIMP NEWBURG

6 ounces fresh *or* frozen shelled shrimp
1 tablespoon butter *or* margarine
5 teaspoons cornstarch
¼ teaspoon salt
1¼ cups skim milk
2 beaten egg yolks
2 tablespoons dry sherry
2 teaspoons lemon juice
3 English muffin halves, toasted

Thaw shrimp if frozen. Halve shrimp lengthwise. In saucepan melt butter; stir in cornstarch and salt. Add milk all at once. Cook and stir till bubbly; cook 2 minutes. Stir *half* of the hot mixture into yolks. Return to hot mixture. Stir in shrimp. Cook and stir about 3 minutes or till bubbly. Cook and stir 1 to 2 minutes more or till shrimp is cooked. Stir in sherry and lemon juice. Spoon over muffin halves. Trim with parsley if desired. Serves 3.

210 BAKED CLAMS AND MUSHROOMS

Serve this entrée for two with a crisp salad—

½ cup sliced fresh mushrooms
¼ cup finely chopped carrot
¼ cup chopped celery
2 tablespoons sliced green onion
⅓ cup skim milk
2 teaspoons cornstarch
¼ teaspoon salt
¼ teaspoon dried rosemary, crushed
1 7½-ounce can minced clams, drained
½ cup shredded process Swiss cheese
Nonstick vegetable spray coating
1 tablespoon fine dry bread crumbs

In a saucepan cook the mushrooms, carrot, celery, and green onion in a small amount of water about 4 minutes or till the vegetables are crisp-tender. Drain. Stir skim milk, the cornstarch, salt, and crushed rosemary together. Stir into the drained vegetables in the saucepan. Cook and stir till mixture is thickened and bubbly. Stir in the drained minced clams and the shredded Swiss cheese. Cook and stir till the cheese is melted and the mixture is heated through.

Spoon clam mixture into two 6-ounce custard cups or individual casseroles that have been sprayed with nonstick vegetable spray coating. Sprinkle mixture in each dish lightly with the dry bread crumbs. Bake in a 400° oven about 10 minutes or till bubbly. Makes 2 servings.

SEASONINGS FOR CALORIE-CUTTERS
Adding a touch of herb to a favorite dish can provide new flavor without furnishing extra calories. When you reduce or omit fat, sugar, or salt from a calorie-trimmed recipe, some flavor is often lost as well. That's where herbs come to the rescue. Use the amount of seasoning suggested in the recipe. Or, if you're creating your own calorie-trimmed recipe, start by using ¼ teaspoon dried herb for each 4 servings.

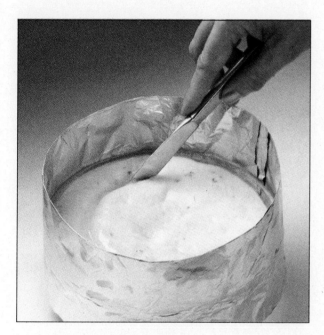

230 BAKED FISH STEAKS

1   **pound halibut, swordfish, *or* salmon steaks,**
    cut 1 inch thick
½   **teaspoon finely shredded lemon peel**
    (set aside)
2   **tablespoons lemon juice**
    Paprika
    Ground red pepper
1   **tablespoon butter *or* margarine**
⅔   **cup plain low-fat yogurt**
¼   **cup shredded cucumber**
2   **tablespoons shredded carrot**
2   **teaspoons snipped chives**
1   **teaspoon sugar**

Place fish on a large piece of heavy-duty foil.
Sprinkle with lemon juice. Sprinkle lightly with
paprika and pepper; dot with butter. Wrap se-
curely; place fish in shallow baking pan. Bake in a
450° oven for 12 to 15 minutes or till fish flakes
easily when tested with a fork. Meanwhile, for the
sauce, in a bowl combine yogurt, cucumber, carrot, chives, sugar, and lemon peel. Garnish fish
steaks with lemon wedges and parsley if desired.
Pass the yogurt sauce with fish. Serves 4.

◄   **TO MAKE A SOUFFLÉ TOP HAT**
After turning the soufflé mixture into a
prepared dish with a collar, use a knife to
trace a one-inch-deep circle through the
mixture as shown. Make the circle about 1
inch from the edge of the dish. As the
soufflé bakes, a "top hat" will form.

247 SHRIMP-SWISS SOUFFLÉ

2   **tablespoons butter *or* margarine**
3   **tablespoons all-purpose flour**
¼   **teaspoon salt**
    Dash pepper
1   **cup skim milk**
1   **cup shredded process Swiss cheese**
4   **egg yolks**
1   **4½-ounce can shrimp, rinsed, drained, and**
    finely chopped
2   **tablespoons snipped parsley**
4   **egg whites**

Attach a foil collar to an *ungreased* 1½-quart
soufflé dish. For the collar, measure enough foil to
go around dish plus a 2- to 3-inch overlap. Fold
foil in thirds lengthwise. Lightly butter one side.
With buttered side in, position foil around outside
of dish, letting collar extend 2 inches above top of
dish; fasten with tape. Set aside.

In saucepan melt butter or margarine; stir in
flour, salt, and pepper. Add milk all at once; cook
and stir over medium heat till thickened and bubbly. Turn heat to low; add Swiss cheese, stirring
till melted. Remove from heat. Cool about 5 minutes while beating egg yolks. In a small mixer
bowl beat egg yolks till thick and lemon-colored.
Slowly add cheese sauce, stirring constantly. Stir
in shrimp and parsley.

Using clean beaters beat egg whites till stiff
peaks form (tips stand straight). Gradually pour
shrimp mixture over egg whites, folding together
thoroughly. Turn mixture into prepared dish. For a
top hat, see tip above. Bake in a 325° oven about
1 hour or till knife inserted near center comes out
clean. Serve immediately. Makes 5 servings.

51

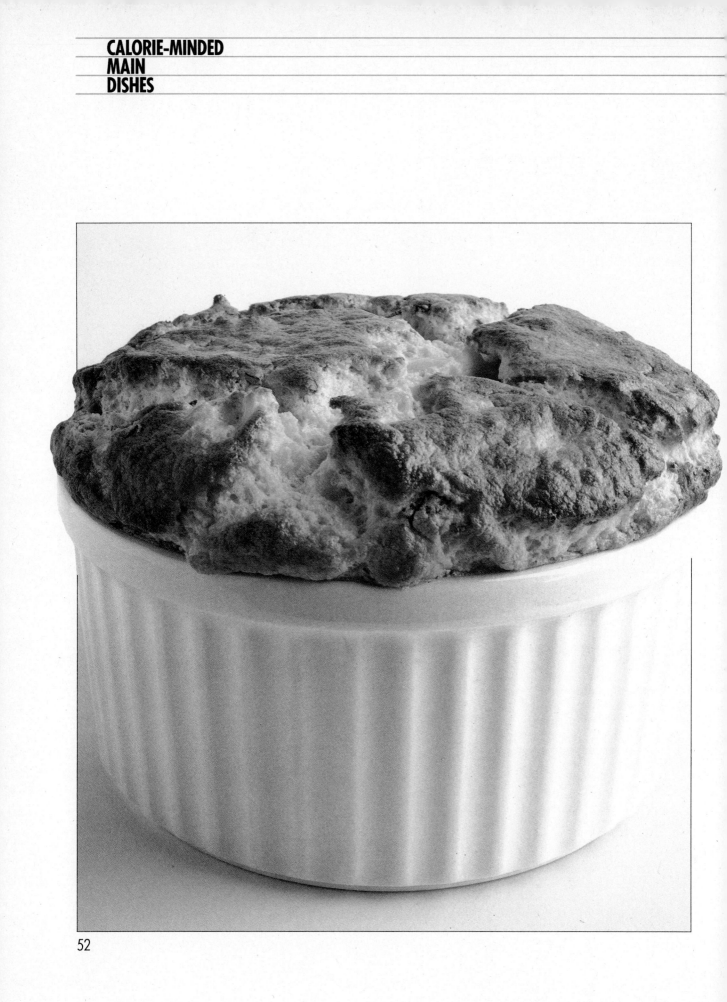

294 BEAN-FILLED OMELET

1 green onion, thinly sliced
½ cup frozen loose-pack French-style
    green beans
¼ cup boiling water
½ cup skim milk
1½ teaspoons cornstarch
2 tablespoons shredded process Swiss
    cheese (½ ounce)
2 eggs
Nonstick vegetable spray coating

Reserve 1 teaspoon green onion. Cook remaining onion and green beans in the ¼ cup boiling water and dash *salt* for about 5 minutes or till tender. Keep warm. In a small saucepan combine the skim milk, cornstarch, ⅛ teaspoon *salt,* and dash *pepper.* Cook and stir till thickened and bubbly. Cook and stir 2 minutes more. Add the cheese; heat and stir till cheese melts. Keep sauce warm while preparing the omelet.

For omelet, in mixing bowl beat eggs, 1 tablespoon *water,* dash *salt,* and dash *pepper* with a fork till blended but not frothy. Spray a 6- or 8-inch skillet with flared sides with nonstick vegetable spray coating. Add egg mixture to prepared skillet; cook over medium heat. As eggs set, run spatula around edge, lifting eggs to allow uncooked portion to flow underneath. When eggs are set but still shiny, remove from heat. Drain heated bean-onion mixture. Stir in 2 tablespoons of the cheese sauce; spoon mixture across center of omelet. Fold one-third of omelet (portion nearest handle of pan) over center; slide toward outside of pan. Fold outer third over filling and slide omelet out onto serving plate. Spoon remaining cheese sauce over. Sprinkle with reserved sliced green onion. Makes 1 serving.

◄ **For a calorie-trimmed luncheon, whip up**
Macaroni-Cheese Puff. **It tastes similar to**
macaroni and cheese but this elegant
version is made puffy with beaten eggs.

---

213 HERBED COTTAGE-SWISS FONDUE

Pictured on page 20—

1 cup low-fat cottage cheese
⅓ cup skim milk
2 tablespoons chopped onion
2 tablespoons snipped parsley
1 tablespoon cornstarch
½ teaspoon dry mustard
½ teaspoon Worcestershire sauce
1 cup shredded process Swiss cheese
2 cups hot crisp-cooked broccoli flowerets
2 cups hot crisp-cooked zucchini chunks
1 cup cherry tomatoes
1 cup fresh mushroom caps

In blender container blend cottage cheese till smooth. Add next 6 ingredients. Cover and blend till smooth. Transfer to saucepan. Cook and stir till bubbly; cook and stir 2 minutes more. Stir in Swiss cheese till melted. Pour into fondue pot; place over fondue burner. Spear vegetables with fondue fork; dip into fondue. Makes 4 servings.

263 MACARONI-CHEESE PUFF

½ cup small elbow macaroni (1¾ ounces)
1½ cups skim milk
1½ cups shredded American cheese (6 ounces)
3 beaten egg yolks
1 cup soft bread crumbs (1⅓ slices)
¼ cup chopped pimiento
2 tablespoons chopped green onion
3 egg whites
¼ teaspoon cream of tartar

Cook macaroni in lightly salted boiling water according to package directions; drain. In saucepan combine milk, cheese, and ¼ teaspoon *salt*; stir over low heat till cheese melts. Stir about *half* of the hot mixture into yolks; return all to saucepan. Stir in macaroni, crumbs, pimiento, and onion. In small mixer bowl beat whites and cream of tartar till stiff peaks form. Fold into macaroni mixture. Bake in *ungreased* 1½-quart soufflé dish in a 325° oven about 1 hour or till knife inserted off-center comes out clean. Serve at once. Serves 5.

53

249 SHIRRED EGGS DELUXE

1 teaspoon butter *or* margarine
4 eggs
Dash pepper
2 teaspoons skim milk
3 tablespoons sliced fresh mushrooms
2 slices bacon, crisp-cooked, drained, and crumbled
2 tablespoons grated Parmesan cheese

Allowing *½ teaspoon* for each, butter 2 shallow individual casseroles. Break 2 eggs into each casserole; add dash pepper. To each casserole add 1 teaspoon milk. Set dishes in an 8x8x2-inch baking pan; place on oven rack. Pour hot water around casseroles to a depth of 1 inch. Bake in a 325° oven for 15 minutes. Top with mushrooms, crumbled bacon, and cheese; return eggs to oven and bake 5 minutes longer. Serves 2.

290 POTATO AND SPINACH SKILLET

Nonstick vegetable spray coating
3 medium potatoes, cooked and shredded
¼ cup chopped onion
¼ cup chopped green pepper
½ teaspoon salt
6 beaten eggs
½ of a 10-ounce package frozen chopped spinach, cooked and well drained
½ cup dry cottage cheese
½ teaspoon celery salt
½ cup shredded American cheese (2 ounces)
1 medium tomato, cut into wedges

Spray a 10-inch skillet with the vegetable spray coating. Combine the potatoes, onion, and green pepper. Pat into skillet. Sprinkle with salt and ⅛ teaspoon *pepper*. Cook, uncovered, over medium heat about 8 minutes. Meanwhile, combine the eggs, spinach, cottage cheese, celery salt, and dash *pepper*; pour atop potatoes. Cover and cook over medium-low heat for 8 to 10 minutes or till almost set. Sprinkle with American cheese. Cook, covered, for 1 to 2 minutes. Garnish with tomato wedges. Makes 4 servings.

270 WHOLE WHEAT MEATLESS PIZZA

Pictured on pages 24 and 25—

¾ cup whole wheat flour
2 tablespoons wheat germ
½ package active dry yeast (1½ teaspoons)
½ teaspoon salt
½ cup warm water (115° to 120°)
2 teaspoons cooking oil
½ to ⅔ cup all-purpose flour
Nonstick vegetable spray coating
1 15-ounce can tomato sauce
2 tablespoons chopped green onion
¾ teaspoon dried oregano, crushed
½ teaspoon dried basil, crushed
⅛ teaspoon garlic powder
4 hard-cooked eggs, sliced
1 medium green pepper, cut into strips
1½ cups shredded mozzarella cheese (6 ounces)

In small mixer bowl combine whole wheat flour, wheat germ, yeast, and salt. Stir in warm water and oil. Beat at low speed with electric mixer for ½ minute, scraping bowl constantly. Beat 3 minutes at high speed. Stir in as much of the all-purpose flour as you can mix in with a spoon. Turn out onto a lightly floured surface. Knead in enough of the remaining all-purpose flour to make a moderately stiff dough that is smooth and elastic (6 to 8 minutes total). Cover the dough and let rest 10 minutes.

On lightly floured surface roll dough into a 13-inch circle; transfer to 12-inch pizza pan that has been sprayed with nonstick vegetable spray coating. Build up edges slightly. Bake in a 425° oven about 12 minutes or till lightly browned.

Meanwhile, combine the tomato sauce, onion, oregano, basil, and garlic powder. Bring to boiling; reduce heat and simmer, uncovered, 5 minutes. If desired, reserve several egg slices for garnish; set aside. Arrange remaining egg slices atop the crust. Spoon tomato mixture over. Top with green pepper. Sprinkle mozzarella cheese atop. Bake in a 425° oven for 10 to 15 minutes longer or till bubbly. Garnish with reserved egg slices. Makes 6 servings.

299 SCRAMBLED EGG-FILLED CREPES

Prepare the Calorie Counter's Crepes the night before so they will be ready to fill and bake for a morning brunch. To store the crepes, stack them between waxed paper, then overwrap the stack before refrigerating. Pictured on pages 10 and 11–

8	Calorie Counter's Crepes (see recipe at right)
8	beaten eggs
¼	cup skim milk
1	tablespoon snipped chives
½	teaspoon salt
1	cup skim milk
1	tablespoon cornstarch
½	teaspoon dry mustard
¼	teaspoon salt
	Dash pepper
¼	cup shredded Monterey Jack cheese (1 ounce)
	Snipped chives

Prepare Calorie Counter's Crepes; set aside. In bowl combine eggs, ¼ cup skim milk, the 1 tablespoon chives, and the ½ teaspoon salt. Pour egg mixture into a 10-inch skillet with a nonstick surface or a skillet sprayed with nonstick vegetable spray coating. Cook eggs over low heat without stirring till mixture begins to set on bottom and around edges. Lift and fold the partially cooked eggs so uncooked portion flows underneath. Continue cooking till eggs are cooked throughout but are still glossy and moist. Remove the eggs from heat immediately.

Place about ¼ cup of the cooked egg along the center of each crepe; fold sides over. Place filled crepes, seam side down, in a 12x7½x2-inch baking dish.

In a saucepan combine the 1 cup skim milk, the cornstarch, dry mustard, ¼ teaspoon salt, and pepper. Cook and stir till thickened and bubbly. Cook and stir 2 minutes more. Stir in the Monterey Jack cheese till melted. Pour sauce over crepes. Bake, covered, in a 375° oven about 15 minutes. Sprinkle the baked crepes with additional snipped chives. Makes 4 servings.

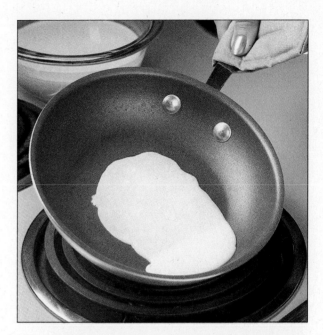

▲ MAKING CALORIE COUNTER'S CREPES
In a bowl combine 1 cup *all-purpose flour*, 1½ cups *skim milk*, 1 *egg*, and ¼ teaspoon *salt;* beat with a rotary beater till blended. Heat a lightly greased 6-inch skillet or a 6-inch skillet sprayed with nonstick vegetable spray coating. Remove the skillet from heat; spoon in about 2 tablespoons batter. Lift and tilt the skillet to spread batter as shown. Return to heat; brown on one side only. Invert pan over paper toweling; remove crepe. Repeat to make about 18 crepes, lightly greasing skillet occasionally. Do not spray the *hot* skillet with nonstick spray coating.

To freeze crepes, stack crepes between layers of waxed paper. Overwrap the stack in a moisture-vaporproof bag, then place in a plastic container. Freeze up to 4 months. Thaw crepes before using. (Each unfilled crepe provides 37 calories.)

CALORIE-MINDED SIDE DISHES

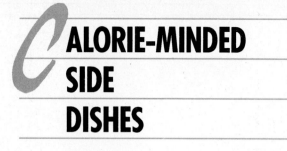

Accompany a meal with side dishes from this chapter. Some tasty examples are those pictured below: Whole Wheat Popovers, Vegetable Bundles with Dairy Dressing, Easy Four-Fruit Salad, and Broccoli-Tomato Stack-Ups (see index for recipe page numbers).

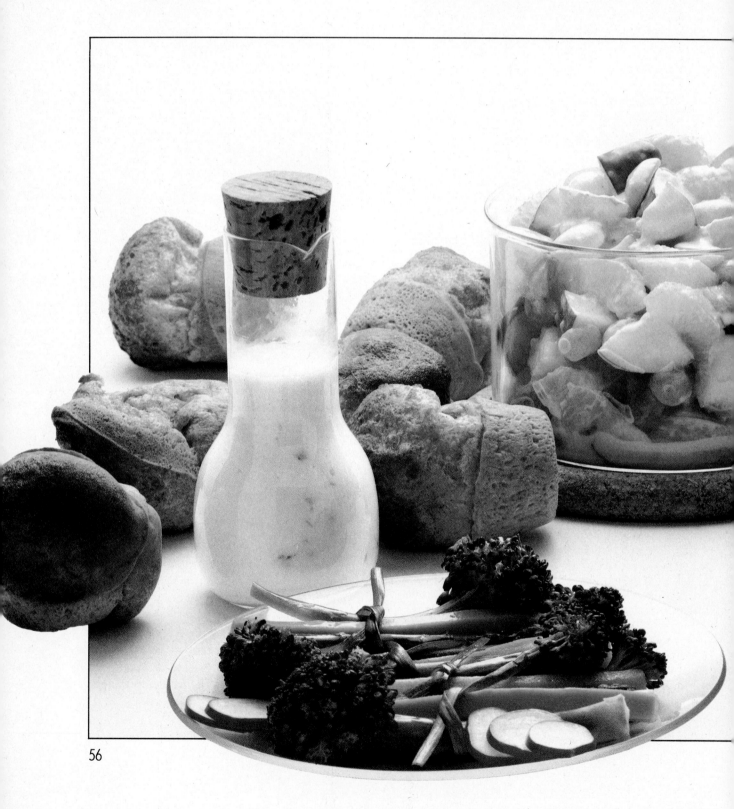

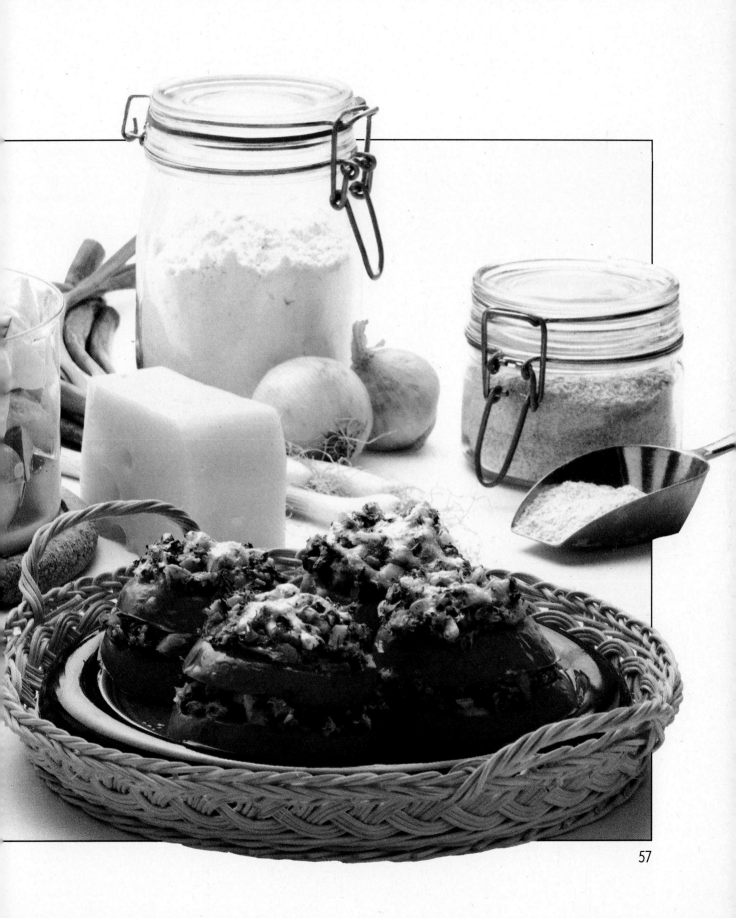

CALORIES PER SERVING		PROTEIN (g)	CARBOHYDRATE (g)	FAT (g)	SODIUM (mg)	POTASSIUM (mg)	PROTEIN	VITAMIN A	VITAMIN C	THIAMINE	RIBOFLAVIN	NIACIN	CALCIUM	IRON
		Per Serving					Percent U.S. RDA Per Serving							
	Breads													
94	Orange-Wheat Muffins (p. 69)	3	15	3	196	77	4	1	9	7	3	4	3	3
119	Quick Garlic Sticks (p. 69)	2	11	8	181	27	4	5	0	5	3	3	3	2
126	Whole Wheat Popovers (p. 69)	6	18	4	181	120	9	0	1	9	11	5	6	3
	Salads and Salad Dressings													
105	Apple-Apricot Salad (p. 66)	2	17	4	32	215	3	15	10	2	3	2	2	5
67	Blueberry-Melon Salad (p. 59)	2	15	0	27	276	3	47	45	4	6	3	6	3
74	Calorie-Trimmed Greek Salad (p. 59)	2	6	5	197	283	3	33	39	4	4	3	7	8
57	Cottage Cheesy Coleslaw (p. 59)	5	6	2	317	198	7	33	48	3	5	1	5	2
114	Curried Winter Fruit Salad (p. 66)	4	21	3	64	435	7	62	47	8	12	3	11	10
11	Diet Russian Dressing (p. 62)	0	3	0	41	23	0	1	1	0	0	0	0	0
67	Easy Four-Fruit Salad (p. 59)	1	15	1	14	163	2	2	23	3	4	1	5	2
16	Gingered Poppy-Seed Dressing (p. 61)	0	4	0	0	28	0	0	11	1	0	0	0	0
96	Mandarin-Pear Salad (p. 66)	2	21	1	28	232	3	7	33	4	6	1	6	3
94	Marinated Potato Salad (p. 67)	3	13	4	39	312	5	6	25	5	5	4	2	6
62	Marinated Vegetable Medley (p. 63)	2	15	0	299	253	3	116	24	3	4	2	5	10
18	Mock Mayonnaise (p. 61)	1	0	1	96	12	2	3	0	1	1	0	1	2
11	Spicy Salad Dressing (p. 62)	0	2	0	72	5	0	0	0	0	0	0	1	0
36	Spinach-Mushroom Salad (p. 59)	3	3	2	139	256	4	49	28	5	9	4	4	8
10	Tofu Dressing (p. 61)	1	1	0	24	20	1	2	1	1	1	0	2	1
101	Vegetable and Cheese Salad (p. 66)	4	15	4	130	246	6	75	19	8	5	5	6	8
34	Vegetable Aspic (p. 62)	3	4	1	136	204	5	21	28	4	3	3	2	4
100	Vegetable Bundles with Dairy Dressing (p. 67)	8	11	3	246	550	12	103	134	12	17	8	10	8
6	Zesty Salad Dressing (p. 61)	0	2	0	64	14	0	1	1	0	0	0	0	0
	Vegetables													
62	Asparagus with Cheese (p. 64)	5	3	4	159	210	8	15	40	9	9	5	11	6
80	Baked Stuffed Potatoes (p. 68)	3	18	0	106	423	4	1	27	6	4	7	3	3
88	Beets and Sweets (p. 69)	2	19	1	196	182	2	92	15	2	2	2	2	4
42	Blender Herbed Tomato Soup (p. 63)	1	6	2	49	222	2	17	28	3	2	4	1	5
70	Broccoli-Tomato Stack-Ups (p. 63)	5	7	3	239	349	8	43	91	6	8	5	11	5
27	Cabbage Scramble (p. 64)	1	6	0	212	200	2	50	39	3	2	1	3	2
35	Cauliflower Italiano (p. 64)	3	6	1	204	324	4	7	122	7	6	4	3	6
95	Celery and Tomatoes au Gratin (p. 68)	5	9	5	449	597	8	18	39	5	8	4	17	5
85	Creamy Asparagus and Carrots (p. 68)	3	6	6	69	258	5	67	34	8	10	5	3	5
74	Hearty Vegetable Soup (p. 63)	3	15	1	524	430	5	100	35	7	7	6	5	7
72	Honey-Glazed Carrot Sticks (p. 64)	1	13	2	114	315	2	201	13	4	3	3	4	4
61	Peas and Onions (p. 64)	4	11	0	188	147	7	12	36	17	5	8	2	9
97	Sprout-Stuffed Tomatoes (p. 68)	4	10	5	159	406	6	28	61	9	7	6	4	7

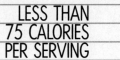
74 CALORIE-TRIMMED GREEK SALAD

⅓ pound romaine, torn (4 cups)
1 cup torn escarole (about 1 ounce)
1 medium tomato
¼ cup sliced cucumber
½ small onion, sliced and separated into rings
3 tablespoons snipped parsley
2 tablespoons crumbled feta cheese (½ ounce)
2 tablespoons sliced pitted ripe olives
3 tablespoons red wine vinegar
1 tablespoon olive oil *or* salad oil
1 tablespoon lemon juice
¼ teaspoon garlic salt
⅛ teaspoon dried oregano, crushed

In a salad bowl combine the torn romaine and escarole. Cut tomato into wedges. Add tomato wedges, cucumber slices, and onion rings to salad greens. Top with parsley, feta cheese, and olives. Cover and chill.

For dressing, in a screw-top jar combine the wine vinegar, olive or salad oil, lemon juice, garlic salt, and oregano. Cover and shake well to mix. Chill thoroughly. Before serving, shake dressing again and pour over salad. Toss to coat vegetables. Makes 4 servings.

67 BLUEBERRY-MELON SALAD

¼ of a cantaloupe, thinly sliced, peeled, and slices halved crosswise
⅓ cup fresh *or* frozen unsweetened blueberries
2 lettuce leaves
¼ cup low-fat pineapple yogurt
¼ teaspoon finely shredded orange peel

Arrange melon pieces and blueberries on two lettuce-lined plates. Drizzle yogurt over fruit. Sprinkle with orange peel. Makes 2 servings.

67 EASY FOUR-FRUIT SALAD

Pictured on pages 56 and 57—

1 cup orange sections (3 medium oranges)
1 cup seedless green grapes, halved
1 cup cubed pear (1 large pear)
1 cup cubed apple (1 large apple)
¾ cup low-fat orange yogurt

In a bowl toss together the orange sections, grapes, pear, and apple. Add the yogurt, tossing gently to coat all the fruit. Cover and chill several hours. If desired, serve on lettuce-lined plates. Makes 8 servings.

36 SPINACH-MUSHROOM SALAD

Pictured on page 23—

1 cup sliced fresh mushrooms
⅓ cup low-calorie Italian salad dressing (no more than 8 calories per tablespoon)
3 cups torn fresh spinach
3 cups torn lettuce
1 hard-cooked egg

Marinate the fresh mushrooms in Italian salad dressing for 1 hour in the refrigerator. In a large salad bowl place spinach, lettuce, and *undrained* mushrooms; toss lightly. Slice egg; arrange over salad. Makes 6 servings.

57 COTTAGE CHEESY COLESLAW

2 cups shredded cabbage
½ cup shredded carrot
2 tablespoons chopped green pepper
½ cup low-fat cottage cheese
2 tablespoons low-calorie creamy cucumber salad dressing

In a bowl toss together first 3 ingredients. In a blender container combine cottage cheese, salad dressing, and ¼ teaspoon *salt*. Cover and blend till smooth. Toss cheese mixture with cabbage mixture till all ingredients are well coated. Cover; chill for several hours. Makes 4 servings.

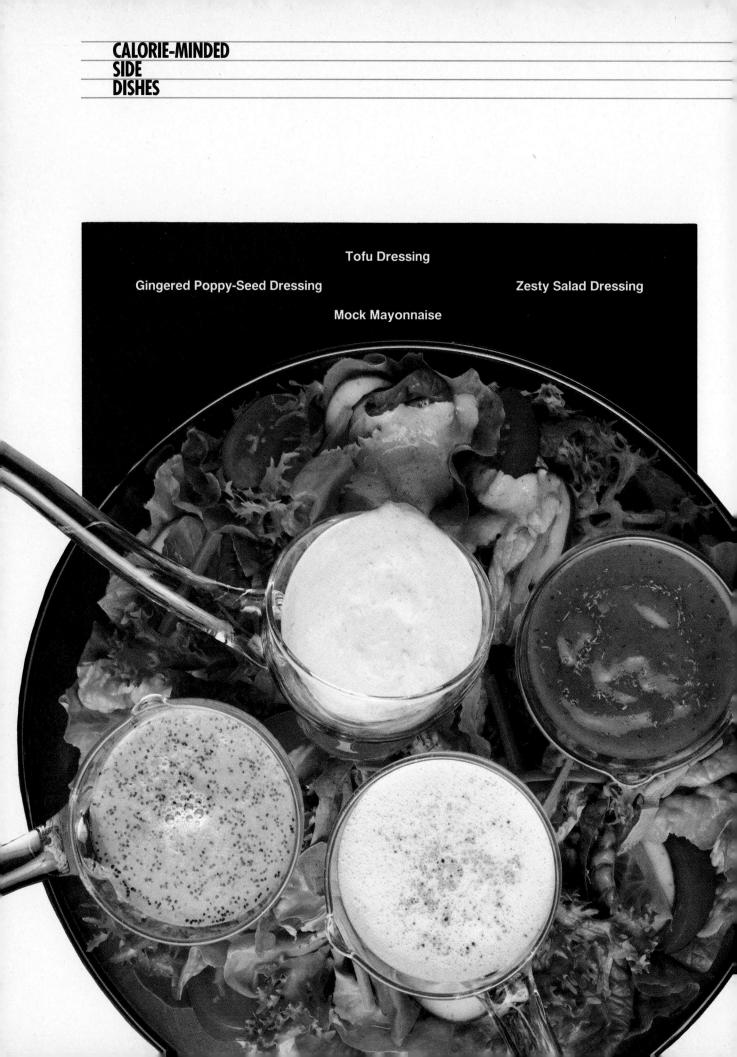

Tofu Dressing

Gingered Poppy-Seed Dressing

Zesty Salad Dressing

Mock Mayonnaise

10 TOFU DRESSING

The flavor is similar to creamy Italian dressing.
Calorie count is for 1 tablespoon of dressing—

8   ounces fresh bean curd (tofu), cubed
1   8-ounce carton plain low-fat yogurt
½   cup chopped fresh spinach
1   tablespoon snipped fresh basil *or* 1
    teaspoon dried basil, crushed
¼   teaspoon salt

In a blender container or food processor bowl place the tofu, yogurt, spinach, basil, and salt. Cover and blend just till smooth. Turn into storage container; cover. Chill dressing thoroughly before serving. Serve with vegetable or main-dish salads. Makes about 1¾ cups dressing.

16 GINGERED POPPY-SEED DRESSING

Calorie count is for 1 tablespoon of dressing—

½   of a 1¾-ounce package (2 tablespoons)
    powdered fruit pectin
1   teaspoon poppy seed
⅛   teaspoon ground ginger
1   cup orange juice
2   tablespoons honey
2   tablespoons lemon juice

In bowl combine pectin, poppy seed, and ginger. Stir in orange juice, honey, and lemon juice. Cover; refrigerate several hours. Stir well before serving. Serve with fruit salads. Makes 1⅓ cups.

◄   **Add flavor to vegetable and fruit salads by spooning on a low-calorie dressing. Select one of the dressings pictured at left or add a bottled low-calorie favorite.**

6 ZESTY SALAD DRESSING

Calorie count is for 1 tablespoon of dressing—

1   tablespoon cornstarch
1   teaspoon sugar
½   teaspoon dried dillweed
¼   teaspoon salt
¼   teaspoon dried basil, crushed
⅛   teaspoon garlic powder
1   cup cold water
¼   cup catsup
3   tablespoons tarragon vinegar *or* cider
    vinegar
1½   teaspoons Worcestershire sauce

In a 1½-quart saucepan combine the cornstarch, sugar, dillweed, salt, basil, and garlic powder. Add water, catsup, vinegar, and Worcestershire sauce. Cook and stir over medium heat till thickened and bubbly; cook and stir 2 minutes more. Cover and chill. Makes 1⅓ cups dressing.

18 MOCK MAYONNAISE

Calorie count is for 1 tablespoon of dressing—

½   teaspoon unflavored gelatin
¼   cup water
3   tablespoons vinegar
2   egg yolks
1   egg
½   teaspoon salt
½   teaspoon sugar
¼   teaspoon dry mustard
¼   teaspoon paprika

In a small saucepan soften gelatin in the water and vinegar; set aside. In a blender container place egg yolks, whole egg, salt, sugar, mustard, and the paprika. Cover and blend about 5 seconds. Bring the gelatin mixture to boiling. With the lid ajar and the blender running at high speed, slowly pour in hot gelatin mixture. Blend about 1 minute. Turn mixture into a bowl; cover and chill several hours. Beat smooth with a rotary beater. Store in refrigerator. Makes ¾ cup dressing.

► **PREPARING VEGETABLE ASPIC**
Pour ½ *cup* of the partially set gelatin mixture into a mold. Arrange egg slices in the mold as shown, pressing eggs gently into gelatin. Carefully spoon the remaining gelatin-vegetable mixture over the layer with egg slices. Chill till firm.

11 DIET RUSSIAN DRESSING

Calorie count is for 1 tablespoon of dressing—

1   1¾-ounce package powdered fruit pectin
1   tablespoon sugar
½   teaspoon dried basil, crushed
¼   teaspoon dried tarragon, crushed
¼   teaspoon garlic salt
¾   cup spicy vegetable juice cocktail
¼   cup wine vinegar

In a bowl combine pectin, sugar, basil, tarragon, and garlic salt. Stir in the vegetable juice cocktail and vinegar. Cover and refrigerate at least 1 hour. Serve on vegetable salads. Makes 1¼ cups.

11 SPICY SALAD DRESSING

Calorie count is for 1 tablespoon of dressing—

2   tablespoons grated Parmesan cheese
1   1¾-ounce package powdered fruit pectin
2   teaspoons sugar
1   teaspoon celery salt
½   teaspoon dried basil, crushed
½   teaspoon dried oregano, crushed
½   teaspoon dry mustard
¼   teaspoon pepper
¼   teaspoon paprika
⅔   cup water
⅓   cup vinegar
1   clove garlic, minced

In a bowl combine the first 9 ingredients. Stir in water, vinegar, and garlic. Cover; refrigerate at least 1 hour. Dressing can be refrigerated for only two to three days. If desired, prepare a half recipe of the dressing at a time. Makes about 1⅓ cups.

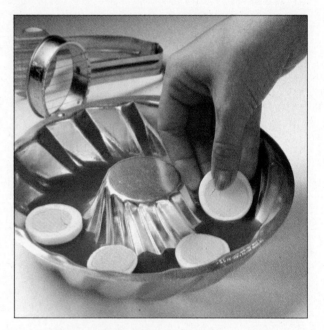

34 VEGETABLE ASPIC

Pictured on page 65—

1   envelope unflavored gelatin
1   12-ounce can (1½ cups) vegetable juice cocktail
2   tablespoons lemon juice
1   hard-cooked egg, sliced
¾   cup cauliflower flowerets, cut up
¼   cup shredded carrot
2   tablespoons sliced green onion

In a small saucepan soften the gelatin in ½ *cup* of the vegetable juice cocktail. Heat and stir till gelatin is dissolved. Stir in the remaining vegetable juice cocktail, lemon juice, and ¼ cup *water*. Chill till the consistency of unbeaten egg whites (partially set). Pour ½ *cup* of the chilled gelatin mixture into a 3-cup ring mold. Press egg slices gently into the gelatin, making a ring in the bottom of the mold. Fold cauliflower, carrot, and onion into remaining gelatin and carefully spoon over the egg slices in bottom of mold. Chill till firm. Unmold onto a plate. Makes 6 servings.

42 BLENDER HERBED TOMATO SOUP

¼ cup chopped onion
2 teaspoons butter *or* margarine
2 cups water
½ of a 6-ounce can tomato paste
1 teaspoon Worcestershire sauce
¼ teaspoon dried basil, crushed
4 thin lemon slices
1 tablespoon snipped parsley

In a saucepan cook the onion in the butter or margarine till tender but not brown. Turn into a blender container. Add the water, tomato paste, Worcestershire sauce, and basil. Cover and blend till smooth. Return mixture to the saucepan. Bring just to boiling. Ladle into bowls. Garnish each serving with a lemon slice and sprinkle with a little of the snipped parsley. Makes 4 servings.

74 HEARTY VEGETABLE SOUP

This is a quick fix-up for canned soup. Be sure to add extra calories if you serve with croutons—

3 cups water
3 medium carrots, sliced (1½ cups)
1 medium onion, chopped
1 16-ounce can stewed tomatoes
1 10¾-ounce can condensed cream of asparagus soup *or* cream of celery soup
1 9-ounce package frozen cut green beans
¼ teaspoon dried oregano, crushed
⅛ teaspoon pepper
Croutons (optional)

In a large saucepan combine water, carrots, onion, *undrained* tomatoes, soup, frozen green beans, oregano, and pepper. Bring to boiling; reduce heat. Cover and simmer about 25 minutes or till beans are tender. If desired, sprinkle individual servings with croutons. Makes 6 servings

70 BROCCOLI-TOMATO STACK-UPS

Pictured on pages 56 and 57—

1 10-ounce package frozen chopped broccoli
3 large tomatoes
½ teaspoon salt
½ cup shredded Monterey Jack *or* Swiss cheese (2 ounces)
2 tablespoons chopped onion

Cook the frozen broccoli according to package directions; drain. Cut each tomato into 4 slices. Sprinkle the tomato slices with the salt and place on the rack of an unheated broiler pan. Combine the broccoli, *2 tablespoons* of the cheese, and the onion. Spoon broccoli mixture atop tomato slices. Broil 4 to 5 inches from heat for 8 to 10 minutes or till hot. Sprinkle with the remaining cheese and broil for 1 to 2 minutes longer or till cheese melts. To serve, stack two tomato slices together, alternating tomato and broccoli layers with cheese on top. Makes 6 servings.

62 MARINATED VEGETABLE MEDLEY

This is a good make-ahead salad—

1 medium cucumber, thinly sliced
1 8-ounce can cut green beans, drained
1 8-ounce can sliced carrots, drained
1 small onion, thinly sliced and separated into rings
½ cup tarragon white wine vinegar
2 tablespoons sugar
¼ teaspoon salt
2 tablespoons snipped parsley

In a bowl combine the cucumber, drained beans, drained carrots, and onion rings. Stir together the vinegar, sugar, and salt till sugar dissolves. Pour over the vegetables. Cover and chill several hours or overnight, stirring occasionally. Before serving, drain off liquid and sprinkle vegetables with the snipped parsley. Makes 4 servings.

72 HONEY-GLAZED CARROT STICKS

5   carrots, cut into julienne strips
      (about 2¼ cups)
1   tablespoon honey
2   teaspoons butter *or* margarine, melted
1   teaspoon prepared mustard
½   teaspoon dried parsley flakes

In a saucepan cook the carrots, covered, in 1 inch of boiling lightly salted water for 10 to 15 minutes or till just tender; drain. Combine honey, butter or margarine, prepared mustard, and dried parsley flakes. Pour honey mixture over the carrots; toss to coat. Makes 4 servings.

27 CABBAGE SCRAMBLE

½   cup water
2   teaspoons instant chicken bouillon granules
3   cups coarsely shredded cabbage
1   cup shredded carrot
1   medium onion, sliced into thin wedges

In a 10-inch skillet combine the water and bouillon granules. Add cabbage, carrot, and onion to the skillet mixture. Cook, covered, over low heat about 15 minutes or till the vegetables are tender. Stir occasionally. Drain the vegetable mixture before serving. Makes 5 servings.

62 ASPARAGUS WITH CHEESE

1   10-ounce package frozen asparagus spears
⅓   cup shredded process Swiss cheese
      (about 1½ ounces)
1   tablespoon chopped pimiento
1½ teaspoons sesame seed, toasted

Cook asparagus spears in boiling lightly salted water according to package directions; drain. Toss together the cheese, pimiento, and sesame seed. Place asparagus in an oven-proof serving dish. Sprinkle cheese mixture over asparagus spears. Heat in a 350° oven about 3 minutes or just till cheese melts. Makes 4 servings.

35 CAULIFLOWER ITALIANO

1   tablespoon chopped onion
1   small clove garlic, minced
2   tablespoons low-calorie Italian salad
      dressing (no more than 8 calories
      per tablespoon)
3   cups small cauliflower flowerets
¼   cup water
1   cup cherry tomatoes, halved
2   tablespoons chopped green pepper
¼   teaspoon salt
⅛   teaspoon dried basil, crushed

In an 8-inch skillet cook onion and garlic in salad dressing till tender; add cauliflower flowerets and water. Cook, covered, over low heat about 15 minutes or till cauliflower is tender. Stir in cherry tomatoes, green pepper, salt, and basil; heat through. Makes 4 servings.

61 PEAS AND ONIONS

Pictured as part of the menu on page 23—

4   green onions
1   16-ounce package frozen peas
2   tablespoons chopped pimiento

Bias-slice the green onions, including the tops, into 1-inch pieces. In a 2-quart saucepan combine the green onion pieces and the frozen peas. Cook vegetables according to package directions for the peas. Drain vegetables. Stir in the chopped pimiento. Makes 6 servings.

▶ **Both of these side dishes add less than 75 calories to your meal. *Asparagus with Cheese* is a frozen vegetable fix-up and *Vegetable Aspic* (see recipe, page 62) is a make-ahead salad.**

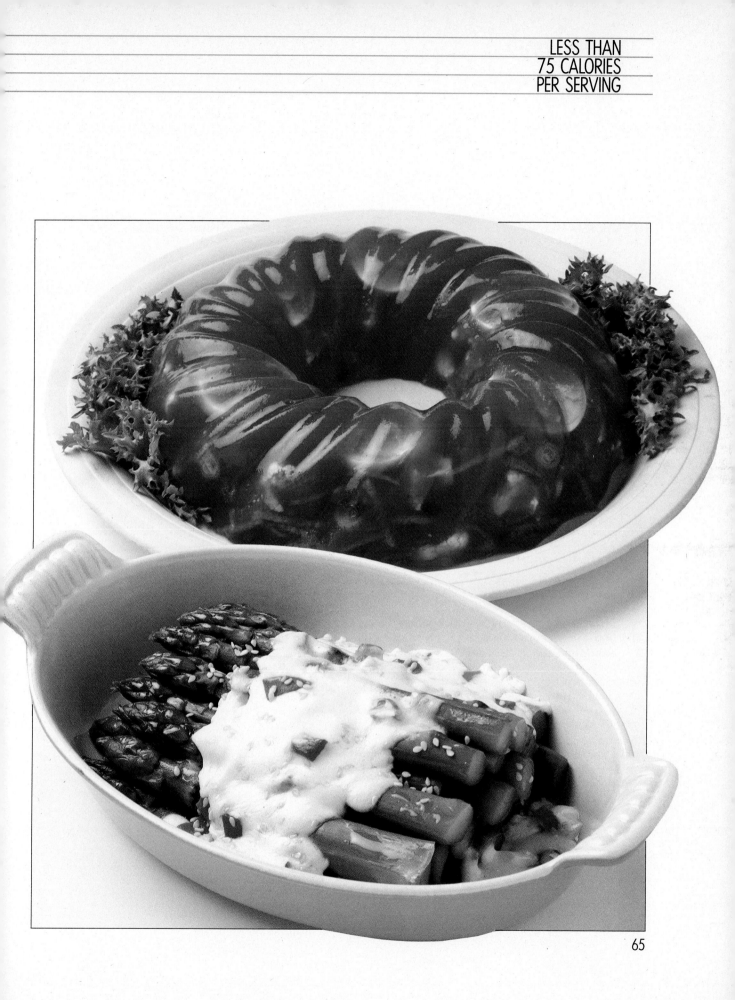

101 VEGETABLE AND CHEESE SALAD

      1 10-ounce package frozen mixed vegetables
    ½ cup sliced zucchini
      2 tablespoons sliced green onion
    ⅓ cup vinegar
      1 tablespoon sugar
      2 teaspoons salad oil
    ⅛ teaspoon garlic salt
      4 lettuce leaves
      2 tablespoons shredded Swiss cheese

Cook frozen vegetables according to package directions; drain. Toss with sliced zucchini and green onion. Combine the vinegar, sugar, oil, and garlic salt. Pour over vegetables. Cover and refrigerate several hours or overnight, stirring occasionally. To serve, spoon drained vegetables onto four individual lettuce-lined plates and sprinkle some of the shredded Swiss cheese atop each serving. Makes 4 servings.

105 APPLE-APRICOT SALAD

      1 envelope unflavored gelatin
      2 cups apple juice
      2 teaspoons lemon juice
      4 fresh apricots, pitted and cut up,
           or 8 canned unpeeled apricot halves
           (water pack), drained and cut up
      1 medium apple, cored and coarsely chopped
      6 lettuce leaves
      2 tablespoons mayonnaise *or* salad dressing

In a saucepan soften the unflavored gelatin in the apple juice. Stir over low heat till gelatin is dissolved. Stir in the lemon juice. Chill till the consistency of unbeaten egg whites (partially set). Fold in the apricots and apple. Turn mixture into six ½-cup molds. Chill till firm. To serve, unmold the salads onto individual lettuce-lined plates. Top each salad with 1 teaspoon of mayonnaise or salad dressing. Makes 6 servings.

114 CURRIED WINTER FRUIT SALAD

      3 tablespoons skim milk
    1½ teaspoons curry powder
      1 8-ounce carton plain low-fat yogurt
      1 tablespoon lemon juice
      2 teaspoons sugar
           Dash ground cinnamon
      4 cups torn fresh spinach *or* lettuce leaves
      2 apples, cored and cut into chunks
      1 pear, cored and cut into chunks
      1 cup fresh alfalfa sprouts
    ½ cup seedless green grapes *or* halved and
           seeded red grapes
    ½ cup sliced celery
      2 tablespoons chopped walnuts

For the dressing, in a small bowl stir together milk and curry powder; let stand a few minutes to moisten spice. Stir in yogurt, lemon juice, sugar, and cinnamon till blended; cover and chill. In a salad bowl toss together spinach, apples, pear, sprouts, grapes, celery, and walnuts. Stir dressing; spoon a little over salad. Pass remaining dressing with salad. Makes 6 servings.

96 MANDARIN-PEAR SALAD

    ⅓ cup plain low-fat yogurt
      1 tablespoon crumbled blue cheese
      1 teaspoon sugar
      2 medium pears, cored and sliced
      1 11-ounce can mandarin orange sections,
           drained
      4 lettuce leaves

In a small bowl stir together yogurt, blue cheese, and sugar. Cover and chill if desired. To prevent pears from darkening, coat with ascorbic acid color keeper prepared according to package directions or with lemon juice mixed with water. Arrange pear slices and mandarin orange sections on four individual lettuce-lined salad plates. Drizzle dressing over salads. Makes 4 servings.

► **MAKING VEGETABLE BUNDLE TIES**

To prepare the green onion ties, cut off green onion tops and slice them lengthwise (as shown) into strips about ¼ inch wide. Immerse strips in boiling water for 1 minute, then drain.

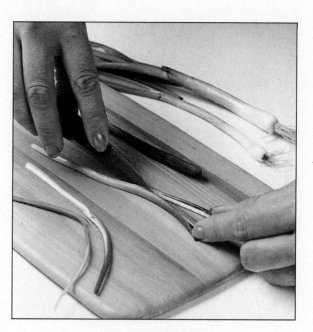

VEGETABLE BUNDLES
100 WITH DAIRY DRESSING

Also pictured on pages 56 and 57—

2	carrots, cut into long thin sticks
8	ounces broccoli, cut into narrow stalks
8	ounces fresh asparagus spears
12	cherry tomatoes
10	radishes
1	or 2 green onions
½	cup low-fat cottage cheese
2	ounces Neufchâtel cheese
1	tablespoon skim milk
1½	teaspoons prepared horseradish
¼	teaspoon onion salt
1	tablespoon chopped pimiento

Place rack in large skillet or Dutch oven. Add water to below rack; bring to boiling. Place carrots on rack. Cover; steam 2 minutes. Add broccoli and asparagus; cover and steam 2 minutes more. Drain. Pour cold water over all vegetables; drain. Wash and drain tomatoes and radishes. Slice radishes, if desired. To make green onion ties for bundles, prepare 10 to 12 strips as described in tip above. Make each strip ¼ inch wide. Immerse strips in boiling water 1 minute; drain on paper toweling.

To assemble bundles, tie an assortment of vegetable strips together carefully with a strip of the green onion. Refrigerate bundles, tomatoes, and radishes till ready to serve.

For dressing, in blender container combine cottage cheese, Neufchâtel cheese, milk, horseradish, and onion salt. Cover; blend till smooth. Add additional skim milk, if necessary, to thin dressing to desired consistency. Stir in pimiento. To serve, arrange bundles, tomatoes, and radishes on plate. Drizzle dressing over vegetables. Makes 5 or 6 servings.

94 MARINATED POTATO SALAD

1	pound potatoes
1	small cucumber, seeded and chopped (1 cup)
½	cup thinly sliced radishes
¼	cup white wine vinegar
¼	cup water
1	tablespoon sugar
½	cup low-sodium mayonnaise
½	teaspoon poppy seed
2	hard-cooked eggs, chopped
8	lettuce leaves

Cook potatoes in boiling water for 25 to 40 minutes or till done. Drain. Cut the potatoes into thick slices. In a large bowl combine cooked potatoes, cucumber, and radishes. Stir together vinegar, water, and sugar; pour over vegetables. Chill the vegetable mixture at least 2 hours.

Drain vegetable mixture thoroughly, reserving 1 tablespoon marinade. Combine mayonnaise, poppy seed, and reserved marinade; pour over potato mixture. Toss to coat. Fold in the chopped hard-cooked eggs. Serve the potato salad in lettuce cups. Makes 8 servings.

CREAMY ASPARAGUS
85 AND CARROTS

¾ pound fresh asparagus, cut up, *or* one
       8-ounce package frozen cut asparagus
2 medium carrots, sliced
1 teaspoon all-purpose flour
    Few dashes ground nutmeg
1 3-ounce package cream cheese, softened
1 tablespoon sliced almonds

In a saucepan cook fresh or frozen asparagus and the carrots, covered, in ½ cup boiling lightly salted *water* about 5 minutes or till just tender. Drain, reserving *⅓ cup* liquid. Return reserved liquid to saucepan. Stir flour and nutmeg into softened cream cheese; add to reserved liquid. Heat and stir over low heat till cheese melts and sauce is bubbly. Gently stir in vegetables; heat through. If desired, season to taste with salt and pepper. Garnish with sliced almonds. Makes 6 servings.

97 SPROUT-STUFFED TOMATOES

4 medium tomatoes
1½ cups fresh bean sprouts
2 tablespoons chopped green onion
1 tablespoon butter *or* margarine
⅛ teaspoon salt
⅓ cup soft whole wheat bread crumbs
1 tablespoon grated Parmesan cheese
2 teaspoons butter *or* margarine, melted

Cut tops off tomatoes; remove centers, leaving shells. Drain tomatoes. Chop enough centers to make ⅓ cup. Cook sprouts and green onion in the 1 tablespoon butter or margarine for 3 to 5 minutes or till tender. Remove from heat; stir in the chopped tomato and the ⅛ teaspoon salt.

Sprinkle insides of tomatoes lightly with salt. Fill tomatoes with sprout mixture. Combine crumbs, cheese, and the 2 teaspoons melted butter or margarine. Sprinkle atop tomatoes. Place tomatoes in an 8x8x2-inch baking pan. Bake in a 375° oven for 20 to 25 minutes or till hot. Serves 4.

80 BAKED STUFFED POTATOES

2 medium baking potatoes
⅓ cup buttermilk
¼ teaspoon seasoned salt
    or butter-flavored salt
1 tablespoon finely chopped green onion
    Paprika

Scrub the potatoes and prick skin with fork. Bake in a 425° oven for 40 to 60 minutes or till done. (Or, wrap each potato in a 6-inch square of heavy-duty foil. Place on a covered grill and lower hood. Grill over *medium-slow* coals for 1½ to 2 hours or till done, turning occasionally. Or, arrange potatoes on paper toweling in a counter-top microwave oven. Micro-cook on high power for 6 to 8 minutes or till done. Halfway through cooking time, rearrange potatoes and turn over.)

Cut baked potatoes in half lengthwise. Reserving potato shells, scoop out the insides and mash. Add buttermilk, seasoned salt, and dash *pepper*; beat till fluffy. Stir in the green onion. Pile lightly into shells. Return to the 425° oven; bake about 10 minutes or till hot. (Or, place on piece of foil in a covered grill and heat about 10 minutes or till hot. Or, place potatoes in nonmetal baking dish and micro-cook, uncovered, on high power about 2 minutes or till potatoes are heated through.) Sprinkle with paprika. Makes 4 servings.

CELERY AND
95 TOMATOES AU GRATIN

1 bunch celery
1 small onion, sliced and separated into rings
2 medium tomatoes, peeled and cut
    into wedges
¾ cup shredded cheddar cheese (3 ounces)

Cut celery stalks into 1-inch pieces (about 7½ cups), reserving tops for another use. In large saucepan cook celery and onion in small amount of boiling water, covered, for 10 to 12 minutes or till celery is crisp-tender. Drain. Stir in tomatoes and ½ teaspoon *salt*; heat through. Turn into a serving dish; top with cheddar cheese. Serves 6.

88 BEETS AND SWEETS

1 8-ounce can small whole sweet potatoes (vacuum pack)
½ cup cold water
1 teaspoon cornstarch
⅛ teaspoon salt
1 tablespoon vinegar
1 teaspoon butter *or* margarine
1 8-ounce can sliced beets, well drained

Slice potatoes; set aside. In a saucepan combine cold water, cornstarch, and salt. Stir in the vinegar and butter or margarine. Cook and stir till mixture is thickened and bubbly. Cook and stir 2 minutes more. Stir in the sweet potato slices and drained beet slices. Cook until heated through. Makes 4 servings.

94 ORANGE-WHEAT MUFFINS

Pictured on page 20—

1 cup whole wheat flour
½ cup all-purpose flour
2 tablespoons sugar
2 teaspoons baking powder
¾ teaspoon salt
1 beaten egg
1 teaspoon finely shredded orange peel
½ cup orange juice
¼ cup skim milk
2 tablespoons cooking oil
Nonstick vegetable spray coating

In a bowl thoroughly stir together the whole wheat flour, all-purpose flour, sugar, baking powder, and salt. Make a well in center of dry ingredients. Combine egg, orange peel, orange juice, milk, and oil. Add all at once to dry ingredients, stirring just till dry ingredients are moistened. Spray 12 muffin cups with nonstick vegetable spray coating. Fill muffin cups about half full with batter. Bake in a 400° oven for 12 to 15 minutes. Store leftover muffins in covered container or wrap and freeze. Reheat muffins before serving. Makes 12.

126 WHOLE WHEAT POPOVERS

Pictured on pages 56 and 57—

1½ teaspoons shortening
3 egg whites
1 cup skim milk
1 tablespoon cooking oil
⅔ cup all-purpose flour
⅓ cup whole wheat flour
½ teaspoon onion salt *or* salt

Grease six 6-ounce custard cups using ¼ *teaspoon* of the shortening for *each* cup. Place custard cups in a 15x10x1-inch baking pan and place in oven. Preheat oven to 450°.

Meanwhile, in 4-cup liquid measure or small mixer bowl combine egg whites, milk, and cooking oil. Add all-purpose flour, whole wheat flour, and onion salt or salt. Beat with rotary beater or electric mixer till mixture is smooth. Remove pan from oven. Fill the hot custard cups *half* full. Return to oven and bake at 450° for 20 minutes. Reduce oven to 350° and bake 15 to 20 minutes more or till popovers are very firm. (If popovers brown too quickly, turn off oven and finish baking in the cooling oven till they are very firm.) A few minutes before removing from oven, prick each popover with a fork to let the steam escape. Serve hot. Makes 6 servings.

119 QUICK GARLIC STICKS

Pictured on pages 10 and 11—

2 frankfurter buns
2 tablespoons butter *or* margarine
1 tablespoon grated Parmesan cheese
¼ teaspoon garlic powder
1 teaspoon sesame seed

Cut each frankfurter bun lengthwise into fourths to make 4 sticks. In a small saucepan heat butter, Parmesan, and garlic powder till butter melts. Brush butter mixture lightly on cut sides of buns using a pastry brush. Sprinkle with sesame seed. Place sticks on baking sheet. Bake in a 375° oven about 10 minutes or till toasted. Serve hot. Makes 4 servings (2 sticks per serving).

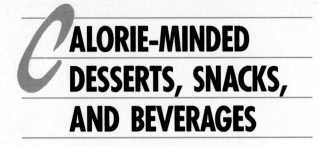

CALORIE-MINDED DESSERTS, SNACKS, AND BEVERAGES

Sometimes a dessert or snack can add a flavor boost to your diet. Try one of the suggestions pictured here: Dilly Cottage Dip, Strawberry Cheese Crepes, Coffee-Cream-Filled Puffs, Apricot-Peach-Filled Puffs, and Fruit Slush (see the index for recipe page numbers).

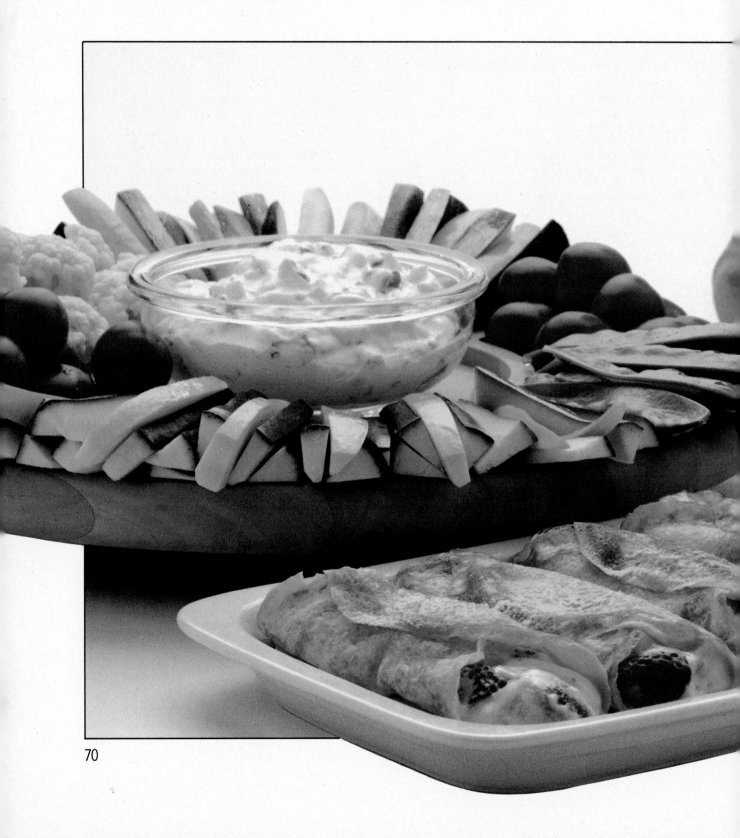

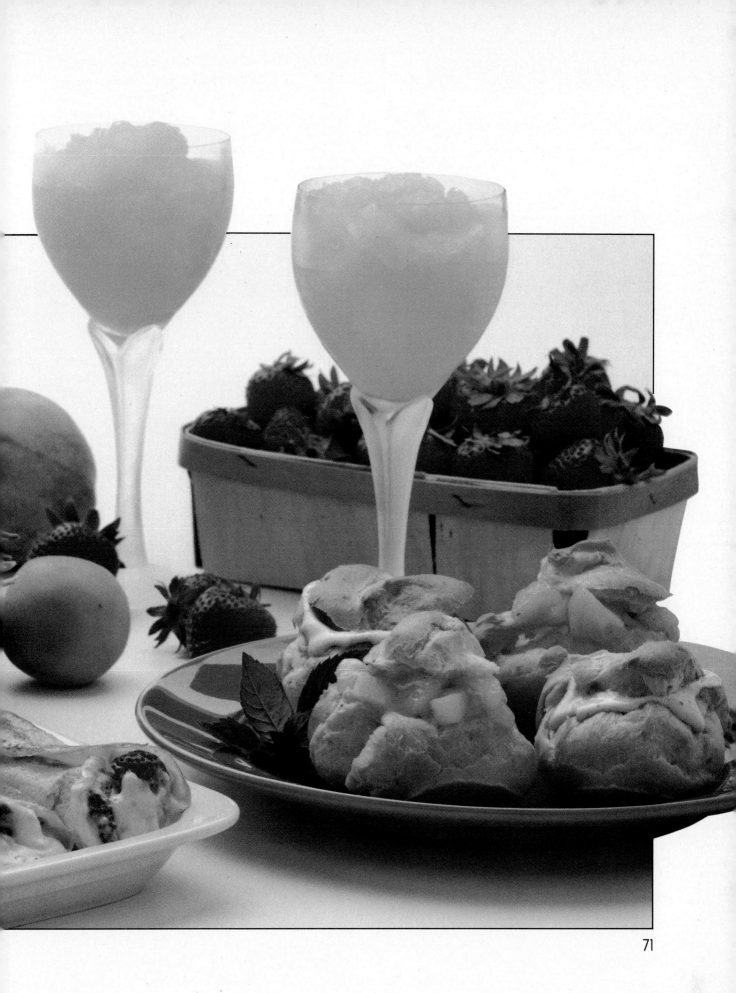

CALORIES PER SERVING		PROTEIN (g)	CARBOHYDRATE (g)	FAT (g)	SODIUM (mg)	POTASSIUM (mg)	PROTEIN	VITAMIN A	VITAMIN C	THIAMINE	RIBOFLAVIN	NIACIN	CALCIUM	IRON
		Per Serving					Percent U.S. RDA Per Serving							
	Desserts													
75	Apple-Berry Dessert (p. 75)	1	19	1	1	150	1	2	21	2	3	2	1	3
68	Apple-Ginger Bake (p. 74)	1	16	1	41	104	1	1	4	3	2	1	1	2
129	Apricot-Peach-Filled Puffs (p. 82)	3	20	5	88	222	5	31	10	5	6	6	2	5
105	Banana Freeze (p. 78)	3	17	3	80	255	5	2	10	3	8	2	8	2
125	Banana Pudding (p. 80)	4	17	5	64	175	6	4	7	3	7	1	5	3
125	Carob Tortoni (p. 78)	2	17	6	117	41	4	0	0	0	3	1	3	1
78	Citrus Special (p. 76)	1	16	2	1	242	2	4	69	5	2	2	3	3
128	Coffee-Cream-Filled Puffs (p. 82)	4	10	8	107	46	6	6	0	4	5	2	1	3
72	Custard-Topped Peaches (p. 75)	3	12	1	47	181	5	15	19	3	7	3	5	2
108	Fluffy Orange Whip (p. 79)	3	18	3	28	58	4	1	2	1	4	0	3	0
79	Four-Fruit Ice (p. 73)	1	19	0	13	105	2	1	30	2	2	1	1	2
61	Frosty Fruit Cup (p. 76)	1	13	0	6	207	1	28	33	5	2	2	2	2
127	Honey Buttermilk Ice Cream (p. 79)	4	20	4	157	151	7	4	4	3	10	1	10	1
91	Lemon-Blueberry Fluff (p. 83)	2	22	0	53	61	3	0	8	1	2	1	0	1
42	Lemony Buttermilk Frappé (p. 75)	3	7	0	106	120	5	0	5	2	9	0	10	0
123	Orange Cheesecake Dessert (p. 79)	4	14	6	75	129	6	6	35	3	5	1	4	0
122	Peaches and Cream Dessert (p. 80)	1	19	4	38	136	2	13	22	4	3	4	1	2
125	Peanut Butter Pops (p. 79)	5	19	4	144	191	8	1	1	3	12	4	13	2
71	Poached Pears (p. 76)	1	17	0	2	155	1	1	10	2	2	1	1	2
76	Pumpkin Chiffon Dessert (p. 73)	4	15	0	172	168	7	53	4	1	6	1	4	2
123	Quick Melon Dessert (p. 80)	3	29	1	44	928	4	30	154	10	7	11	5	8
88	Raspberry Ice (p. 78)	1	22	0	28	79	2	1	22	1	2	2	1	2
73	Raspberry-Yogurt Dessert (p. 73)	2	15	1	36	113	3	1	17	2	7	2	5	2
78	Rhubarb-Strawberry Bowl (p. 73)	1	19	0	2	200	1	2	51	2	4	2	6	4
79	Spicy Peach Compote (p. 74)	1	20	0	1	239	1	20	22	4	3	5	1	3
74	Strawberries Juliet (p. 75)	1	13	2	10	180	2	2	92	2	6	3	4	5
129	Strawberry Cheese Crepes (p. 83)	5	18	4	121	160	8	4	19	5	11	3	10	3
115	Strawberry-Flavored Yogurt (p. 83)	5	18	3	77	256	8	2	27	5	17	2	19	1
62	Strawberry-Glazed Melon Balls (p. 76)	1	15	0	10	245	1	55	70	3	2	3	2	3
116	Tropical Cantaloupe Frost (p. 80)	3	21	3	40	199	4	30	25	3	8	2	9	1
79	Yogurt-Fruit Medley (p. 74)	1	19	1	9	215	2	3	47	6	4	2	4	2
	Snacks and Beverages													
60	Apple-Cot Cooler (p. 87)	0	15	0	1	154	1	9	15	1	1	1	1	3
79	Breakfast Mocha Cocoa (p. 87)	7	13	1	88	298	10	0	3	4	19	2	21	2
46	Cottage Cheese-Deviled Eggs (p. 86)	4	1	3	100	42	6	6	1	2	5	0	2	4
16	Dilly Cottage Dip (p. 84)	2	1	1	97	21	3	1	2	0	1	0	1	0
71	Fruit Slush (p. 87)	0	19	0	1	26	0	0	18	1	1	1	0	0
67	Hot Fruity Spiced Tea (p. 87)	1	16	0	1	229	1	3	62	6	2	2	2	2
60	Pickled Shrimp (p. 86)	11	3	0	214	162	17	1	3	1	1	9	4	6
67	Strawberry Shake (p. 87)	3	14	0	39	205	5	1	60	3	10	2	10	3
76	Taco Popcorn Snack (p. 84)	1	11	3	131	24	2	14	6	9	9	6	1	15
15	Tuna Balls (p. 84)	1	0	1	28	17	2	2	1	0	1	2	0	0
12	Zesty Vegetable Dip (p. 86)	1	2	1	23	18	1	1	4	1	1	1	1	1
24	Zucchini Dip (p. 84)	1	1	2	60	38	1	3	4	1	2	1	1	0

79 FOUR-FRUIT ICE

1	fully ripe medium banana, mashed
½	teaspoon finely shredded orange peel
½	cup orange juice
1	tablespoon lemon juice
1½	cups cranberry juice cocktail
¼	cup sugar
2	stiff-beaten egg whites

In a mixing bowl combine banana, orange peel, orange juice, and lemon juice. Beat till smooth. Stir in cranberry juice cocktail and sugar. Turn into an 8x4x2-inch loaf pan; freeze till firm. Break frozen mixture into chunks in a chilled mixer bowl. Using chilled beaters, beat with an electric mixer till smooth. Return to pan. Freeze till firm. Beat mixture in chilled mixer bowl a second time, then fold in the stiff-beaten egg whites. Return to pan and freeze till firm. Let stand a few minutes before scooping into dessert dishes. Makes 8 servings.

78 RHUBARB-STRAWBERRY BOWL

Pictured on pages 10 and 11—

¼	cup water
¼	cup sugar
8	ounces fresh or frozen rhubarb, cut into 1-inch pieces (about 2 cups)
2	tablespoons orange juice
2	teaspoons cornstarch
1	cup fresh strawberries, sliced

In a 1-quart saucepan combine the water and sugar. Bring to boiling; add the rhubarb. Reduce heat; cover and simmer about 2 minutes or till rhubarb is almost tender. Remove from heat. Drain, reserving the syrup. Add water to reserved syrup, if necessary, to make ¾ cup liquid. Mix the orange juice and cornstarch. Add to the ¾ cup syrup mixture in saucepan. Cook and stir till thickened and bubbly. Cook and stir 2 minutes more. Remove from heat and cool slightly. Gently stir in the rhubarb and strawberries. Chill. To serve, spoon into dessert dishes. Makes 4 servings.

73 RASPBERRY-YOGURT DESSERT

1	10-ounce package frozen red raspberries
1	tablespoon cornstarch
1	8-ounce carton plain low-fat yogurt
¼	teaspoon almond extract
1	egg white
¼	teaspoon cream of tartar

Thaw raspberries; drain, reserving syrup. Add water to syrup to make 1 cup. In a saucepan stir syrup mixture into cornstarch. Cook and stir over medium heat till thickened and bubbly. Cook and stir 2 minutes more. Remove from heat; cover surface. Cool to room temperature without stirring. Stir in the yogurt and extract. Fold in raspberries. Beat egg white and cream of tartar till stiff peaks form (tips stand straight). Gently fold into yogurt mixture. Spoon into dessert dishes. Chill. Makes 6 servings.

76 PUMPKIN CHIFFON DESSERT

2	tablespoons brown sugar
1	envelope unflavored gelatin
¼	teaspoon salt
¼	teaspoon pumpkin pie spice
⅓	cup skim milk
¼	cup water
⅔	cup canned pumpkin
2	egg whites
2	tablespoons sugar
	Mint sprigs or orange peel curls (optional)

In a saucepan combine the brown sugar, gelatin, salt, and pumpkin pie spice. Stir in the milk and water. Heat and stir till gelatin is dissolved. Remove from heat. Stir in the pumpkin. Chill till partially set, stirring occasionally. In small mixing bowl beat egg whites to soft peaks (tips curl over); gradually add the sugar, beating till stiff peaks form (peaks stand straight). Fold into pumpkin mixture. If necessary, chill the mixture till it mounds. Spoon pumpkin mixture into dessert dishes. Chill. Garnish with mint sprigs or orange peel if desired. Makes 4 servings.

79 YOGURT-FRUIT MEDLEY

2 teaspoons sugar
2 teaspoons cornstarch
½ cup unsweetened pineapple juice
½ teaspoon vanilla
½ cup plain low-fat yogurt
3 medium oranges, peeled, sectioned, and coarsely chopped
2 medium apples, cored and thinly sliced
1 cup seedless green grapes, halved

In a small saucepan combine the sugar and cornstarch. Stir in pineapple juice. Stir over medium heat till thickened and bubbly. Cook and stir 2 minutes more. Remove from heat; stir in vanilla. Cool 10 minutes without stirring. Stir mixture into yogurt. Add oranges, apples, and grapes. Mix lightly. Cover; chill. Serve in dishes. Serves 8.

79 SPICY PEACH COMPOTE

2 large or 4 small fresh peaches
4 teaspoons sugar
1 teaspoon cornstarch
½ cup water
¼ cup frozen pineapple-orange juice concentrate, thawed
¼ teaspoon finely shredded orange peel
4 inches stick cinnamon
3 whole cloves

Peel, halve, and pit peaches. To prevent peaches from darkening, coat with ascorbic acid color keeper prepared according to package directions or coat with lemon juice mixed with water.

In a medium saucepan mix sugar and cornstarch. Stir in water, thawed pineapple-orange juice concentrate, orange peel, cinnamon, and cloves. Cook and stir till mixture is thickened and bubbly; cook and stir 2 minutes more. Place peaches in sauce mixture, turning peaches to coat. Cover and simmer 2 to 3 minutes; remove from heat. Transfer to bowl; cover and chill. Remove spices before serving. Makes 4 servings.

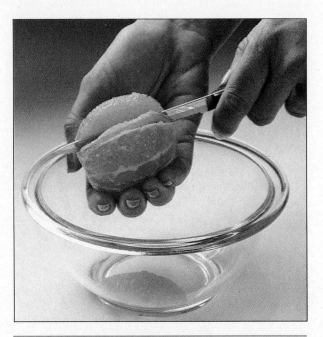

▲ **SECTIONING CITRUS FRUIT**
Remove the peel and white membrane using a very sharp utility knife or serrated knife. To remove sections, cut into the center of the fruit between one section and the membrane as shown. Then turn the knife and slide it down the other side of the section next to the membrane. Work over a bowl to catch the juice.

68 APPLE-GINGER BAKE

2 tablespoons water
1 teaspoon brown sugar
1 teaspoon lemon juice
1 cup sliced, peeled apples
2 gingersnap cookies, crushed

Combine water, brown sugar, and lemon juice; mix with the apples. Divide the apple mixture between two 6-ounce custard cups. Cover with foil. Bake in a 375° oven for 20 minutes. Uncover and sprinkle with crushed gingersnap cookies. Bake 5 minutes more. Serve warm. Makes 2 servings.

72 CUSTARD-TOPPED PEACHES

1 cup skim milk
2 slightly beaten egg yolks
2 tablespoons sugar
½ teaspoon vanilla
2 tablespoons frozen orange juice
   concentrate, thawed
½ teaspoon finely shredded lemon peel
4 fresh peaches *or* two 16-ounce cans
   calorie-reduced peach slices
2 egg whites
¼ teaspoon vanilla
1 tablespoon sugar

For custard mixture, in a small saucepan combine skim milk, egg yolks, 2 tablespoons sugar, and dash *salt*. Cook and stir over medium heat till mixture just comes to boiling. Stir in the ½ teaspoon vanilla. Chill mixture quickly by placing in bowl of ice water. Stir orange juice concentrate and lemon peel into chilled custard mixture.

Peel, pit, and slice fresh peaches or drain canned peaches. Divide peaches among eight 6-ounce custard cups. Spoon custard mixture atop peaches. Beat egg whites and ¼ teaspoon vanilla till soft peaks form (tips curl over). Gradually add 1 tablespoon sugar; beat till stiff peaks form (tips stand straight). Dollop meringue atop mixture in custard cups. Bake in a 400° oven 6 to 8 minutes or till meringue is lightly browned. Serve warm. Makes 8 servings.

74 STRAWBERRIES JULIET

2½ cups hulled fresh strawberries, halved
⅓ cup frozen whipped dessert topping,
   thawed
⅓ cup plain low-fat yogurt
1 tablespoon sugar

Crush ¼ *cup* of the strawberries. Combine the crushed berries, thawed dessert topping, yogurt, and sugar. Spoon halved berries into 4 sherbet glasses. Top with yogurt mixture. Serves 4.

LOW-CAL SUBSTITUTES
You'll often find that it works just as well to use a low-calorie option in place of a high-calorie food. Compare these foods:
- **One cup of sweetened applesauce has 232 calories and one cup of unsweetened applesauce has 100.**
- **One cup of dairy sour cream has 493 calories and one cup of plain low-fat yogurt contains only 123 calories.**
- **One cup of vanilla ice cream has 257 calories but the same amount of vanilla ice milk has 199.**

42 LEMONY BUTTERMILK FRAPPÉ

1⅓ cups buttermilk
1 tablespoon sugar
½ teaspoon finely shredded lemon peel
1 tablespoon lemon juice
1 cup ice cubes
   Ground nutmeg

In a blender container combine buttermilk, sugar, lemon peel, and lemon juice. Add ice cubes, one at a time, blending till crushed. Pour into four chilled glasses. Sprinkle each serving with a dash of nutmeg. Serve immediately. Makes 4 servings.

75 APPLE-BERRY DESSERT

Prepare with either raspberries or blueberries—

3 tablespoons unsweetened pineapple juice
2 teaspoons honey
2 teaspoons lemon juice
⅛ teaspoon ground cinnamon
2 medium apples
1 cup fresh red raspberries *or* blueberries

In a small bowl combine the pineapple juice, honey, lemon juice, and cinnamon. Core and cut apples into thin wedges. Toss apple wedges and berries with the juice mixture. Serve in dessert dishes. Makes 4 servings.

61 FROSTY FRUIT CUP

1 15¼-ounce can pineapple chunks
     (juice pack)
1 16-ounce bottle low-calorie lemon-lime
     carbonated beverage
2 tablespoons lime juice
     Few drops green food coloring (optional)
2 cups cantaloupe balls
1 cup seedless green grapes
     Fresh mint sprigs (optional)

Drain pineapple, reserving juice. In a bowl combine pineapple juice, carbonated beverage, lime juice, and food coloring if desired; stir. Pour into a 9x5x3-inch or an 8x4x2-inch loaf pan; freeze 2 to 2½ hours or just till mixture is slushy. In a bowl combine pineapple chunks, cantaloupe balls, and grapes. Spoon fruit into eight sherbet dishes; top with slush. Trim with fresh mint sprigs if desired. Makes 8 servings.

62 STRAWBERRY-GLAZED MELON BALLS

1 cup fresh strawberries
½ cup water
3 tablespoons sugar
1 tablespoon cornstarch
1 tablespoon lemon juice
3 cups cantaloupe balls
     or honeydew melon balls

In a saucepan crush strawberries; add the water. Bring to boiling; reduce heat. Cover and simmer 5 minutes. Sieve. Return berry juice to saucepan. Combine the sugar and cornstarch; stir into berry juice. Cook and stir till mixture is thickened and bubbly. Cook and stir 2 minutes more. Stir in lemon juice. Cover surface with waxed paper and cool 45 minutes. Spoon melon balls into six dessert dishes. Drizzle strawberry mixture over the melon balls. Chill. Makes 6 servings.

78 CITRUS SPECIAL

1 cup orange sections
1 small banana, sliced
½ cup grapefruit sections
1 tablespoon frozen orange juice concentrate,
     thawed
⅓ cup frozen whipped dessert topping,
     thawed

Combine the orange, banana, and grapefruit; spoon into four dessert dishes. Chill. In a small bowl fold orange juice concentrate into topping. Before serving, dollop topping on fruit. Garnish with fresh mint sprigs if desired. Serves 4.

71 POACHED PEARS

3 medium pears
     Ascorbic acid color keeper
1 6-ounce can unsweetened pineapple juice
1 tablespoon orange liqueur
     Fresh mint sprigs (optional)

Peel, halve, and core pears; dip in ascorbic acid color keeper prepared according to package directions. In skillet bring pineapple juice to boiling; add pears. Reduce heat; simmer, covered, for 10 to 20 minutes or till pears are tender, stirring occasionally. Stir liqueur into liquid in skillet. If pears are very firm and take longer to cook, it may be necessary to stir 2 tablespoons *water* into liquid in skillet before serving. Spoon fruit and syrup into dishes. Trim with mint if desired. Serves 6.

▶ **Fresh and juice-pack canned fruits are good choices for diet desserts. Two recipes using fruits are *Poached Pears* and *Frosty Fruit Cup*. The fruit cup has three fruits topped with an icy slush.**

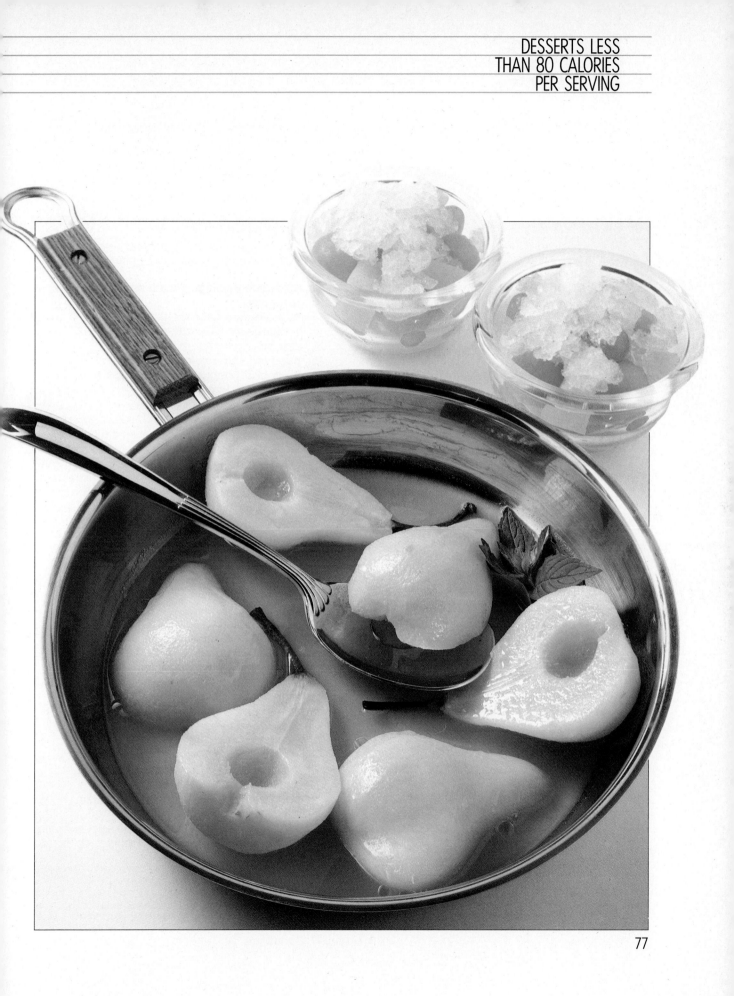

105 BANANA FREEZE

Pictured on pages 10 and 11—

1   cup buttermilk
¾   cup mashed fully ripe banana
½   cup frozen whipped dessert topping, thawed
1½ teaspoons finely shredded orange peel
2   tablespoons shredded coconut, toasted

Pour buttermilk into a shallow container; freeze till ice crystals form around edges (about 30 minutes). In a chilled bowl whip the buttermilk with electric mixer till fluffy. Fold in the banana, topping, and orange peel. Pour into an 8x4x2-inch loaf pan. Cover and freeze till firm. Let stand at room temperature 20 minutes before scooping. Sprinkle with toasted coconut. Makes 4 servings.

LOW-CALORIE GARNISHES

Perk up the appearance of your calorie-trimmed foods with an attractive garnish:

● **Consider the container in which you serve the food and the accessories. An elegant stemmed glass does wonders for a small dessert portion. Colorful straws make a low-cal beverage appear special.**

● **Arrange lemon or orange slices on the plate with fresh parsley or mint sprigs. Sprinkle shredded peel atop a dessert.**

● **Strawberries add color to a dessert. Use whole berries, with or without the hulls, or arrange sliced berries atop the food.**

● **Other fruit trims include melon balls, apple or pear wedges, pineapple chunks, and orange or tangerine sections.**

● **Sprinkle ground spice on a dessert or paprika on a main dish for color.**

● **Carrots make a colorful trim. Form them into curls, or cut them into julienne strips.**

● **Other vegetable garnishes include cucumber slices, pimiento, green pepper rings, radishes, and cherry tomatoes.**

88 RASPBERRY ICE

This dessert can be made year round because frozen raspberries are used for the fruity base—

1   10-ounce package frozen red raspberries, thawed
½   of a 3-ounce package (about ¼ cup) raspberry-flavored gelatin
½   cup boiling water
½   cup cold water
¼   teaspoon finely shredded lemon peel
1   tablespoon lemon juice

Sieve the raspberries; discard seeds. Set sieved berries aside. Dissolve gelatin in the boiling water. Stir in the cold water, lemon peel, and lemon juice. Stir in the sieved berries. Pour mixture into an 8x4x2-inch loaf pan and freeze for 3 to 4 hours or till mixture is firm. Break into chunks and place in a chilled bowl. Beat mixture with an electric mixer till smooth. Return to loaf pan and freeze about 2 hours or till firm. Makes 5 servings.

125 CAROB TORTONI

1   egg white
⅛   teaspoon salt
⅛   teaspoon cream of tartar
1   tablespoon sugar
2   tablespoons carob powder
4   large maraschino cherries, chopped
1   tablespoon chopped almonds
½   of a 4-ounce container (scant 1 cup) frozen whipped dessert topping, thawed

In a small bowl beat egg white, salt, and cream of tartar till soft peaks form (tips curl over). Gradually add the sugar, beating till stiff peaks form (peaks stand straight). Fold egg white, carob powder, cherries, and almonds into the thawed topping. Turn mixture into 3 paper bake cups in muffin pans. Freeze till firm. Remove paper cups before serving. Makes 3 servings.

125 PEANUT BUTTER POPS

1 4-serving-size package *regular* vanilla
   pudding mix
2 cups skim milk
1 5⅓-ounce can (⅔ cup) evaporated milk
2 tablespoons peanut butter

Prepare vanilla pudding according to package directions, *except* use the 2 cups skim milk and the evaporated milk. Remove from heat and stir in the peanut butter till melted. Cool 5 minutes, stirring twice. Pour into a pan and freeze till ice crystals form around edges of pan. Turn into a chilled bowl and beat till smooth. Pour mixture into eight 3-ounce paper drink cups. Insert a wooden stick into each. Freeze till mixture is firm. To serve, peel off the paper cups. Makes 8 servings.

123 ORANGE CHEESECAKE DESSERT

Pictured on page 23—

2 tablespoons sugar
1 envelope unflavored gelatin
½ teaspoon finely shredded orange peel
1 cup orange juice
3 ounces Neufchâtel cheese, cut up
1 teaspoon vanilla
1 1¼-ounce envelope dessert topping mix
½ cup skim milk
   Orange peel (optional)

In a saucepan combine the sugar and unflavored gelatin. Set the ½ teaspoon shredded orange peel aside. Stir orange juice into gelatin mixture. Stir over low heat till gelatin is dissolved. Pour into a blender container. Add the cut up cheese and vanilla. Cover and blend till mixture is smooth. Stir in the orange peel. Chill till mixture is the consistency of unbeaten egg whites (partially set).

Meanwhile, in a mixing bowl prepare the dessert topping mix according to package directions, *except* use the skim milk. Fold cheese mixture into topping. Spoon mixture into .six stemmed sherbet dishes. Cover and chill. To serve, top each serving with additional shredded orange peel if desired. Makes 6 servings.

127 HONEY BUTTERMILK ICE CREAM

1 8-ounce package Neufchâtel cheese,
   softened
⅔ cup honey
1 quart buttermilk (4 cups)
1 cup unsweetened pineapple juice
1 teaspoon vanilla

In a bowl combine the cheese and honey; beat till smooth and creamy. Stir in the buttermilk, pineapple juice, and vanilla. Pour into an ice cream freezer container; freeze according to freezer manufacturer's directions. Serve with fresh fruit if desired. Makes about 14 half-cup servings.

108 FLUFFY ORANGE WHIP

You can make up to 8 servings from this recipe. Each serving then adds 81 calories to the diet—

⅓ cup sugar
½ of an envelope (about 1¼ teaspoons)
   unflavored gelatin
⅔ cup water
2 egg whites
¼ teaspoon finely shredded orange peel
1 tablespoon orange juice
¼ teaspoon vanilla
1 cup frozen whipped dessert topping,
   thawed
½ cup low-fat orange yogurt
   Ground nutmeg *or* ground cinnamon
   Finely shredded orange peel (optional)

In saucepan combine sugar and gelatin. Stir in water. Stir over medium heat till gelatin dissolves. Chill till the consistency of unbeaten egg whites (partially set). Add egg whites, the ¼ teaspoon orange peel, orange juice, and vanilla. Beat with an electric mixer at high speed 4 to 5 minutes or till very fluffy. If necessary, chill till partially set. Fold in the dessert topping and orange yogurt. Pile mixture into six dessert dishes. Sprinkle lightly with nutmeg and garnish with orange peel if desired. Chill till firm. Makes 6 servings.

79

116 TROPICAL CANTALOUPE FROST

This frothy summer dessert-in-a-glass has a delightful fruit flavor—

2 cups cubed cantaloupe *or* honeydew melon
      (½ of a medium melon)
2 cups cold milk
¼ teaspoon ground ginger
1 pint orange sherbet
   Orange peel curls (optional)

Place melon cubes in a freezer-proof bowl and put in the freezer. Freeze till firm. In a blender container or food processor bowl combine frozen melon cubes, milk, and ginger; blend till slushy. Add sherbet a spoonful at a time, blending till thoroughly mixed and stopping to scrape sides of blender as necessary. Pour into eight chilled glasses. Garnish each glass with an orange peel curl if desired. Makes 8 servings.

125 BANANA PUDDING

2 tablespoons sugar
½ of an envelope (about 1¼ teaspoons)
      unflavored gelatin
½ cup skim milk
1 beaten egg
1 ripe medium banana
2 teaspoons lemon juice
¾ cup frozen whipped dessert topping,
      thawed

In a saucepan combine the sugar, gelatin, and dash *salt*. Stir in the skim milk. Stir over medium heat till gelatin is dissolved. Stir about *half* of the hot mixture into the beaten egg; return to hot mixture in saucepan. Cook and stir 1 to 2 minutes more. Chill till consistency of unbeaten egg whites (partially set). Mash banana; add lemon juice. Stir into gelatin mixture. Fold whipped topping into the banana mixture. Spoon into four dessert dishes. Chill till firm. Garnish with sprigs of fresh mint if desired. Makes 4 servings.

122 PEACHES AND CREAM DESSERT

18 vanilla wafers
 1 1¼-ounce envelope dessert topping mix
½ cup orange juice
1½ cups fresh *or* frozen unsweetened
       sliced peaches
⅛ teaspoon ground nutmeg

Line six dessert dishes using 3 vanilla wafers for each dish. Prepare dessert topping mix according to package directions, *except* use the orange juice instead of the milk. Thaw peaches, if frozen, and drain. Chop peaches coarsely. Fold fresh or thawed peaches and nutmeg into the whipped topping. Spoon peach mixture into the cookie-lined dessert dishes. Cover and chill. If desired, garnish each serving with shredded orange peel. Makes 6 servings.

123 QUICK MELON DESSERT

1 small honeydew melon (4½ pounds)
2 tablespoons orange juice
2 teaspoons lime juice
1 cup cantaloupe balls

Cut honeydew melon into quarters. Remove and discard seeds. Place melon wedges on serving plates. Drizzle a mixture of the orange juice and lime juice over cantaloupe balls. Spoon melon balls and juice into melon wedges. Garnish with fresh mint sprigs if desired. Makes 4 servings.

► **When melons are in season, plan either of these recipes for dessert.** *Tropical Cantaloupe Frost* **is a snap to make in the blender and** *Quick Melon Dessert* **is a simple, dressed up way to serve the fruit.**

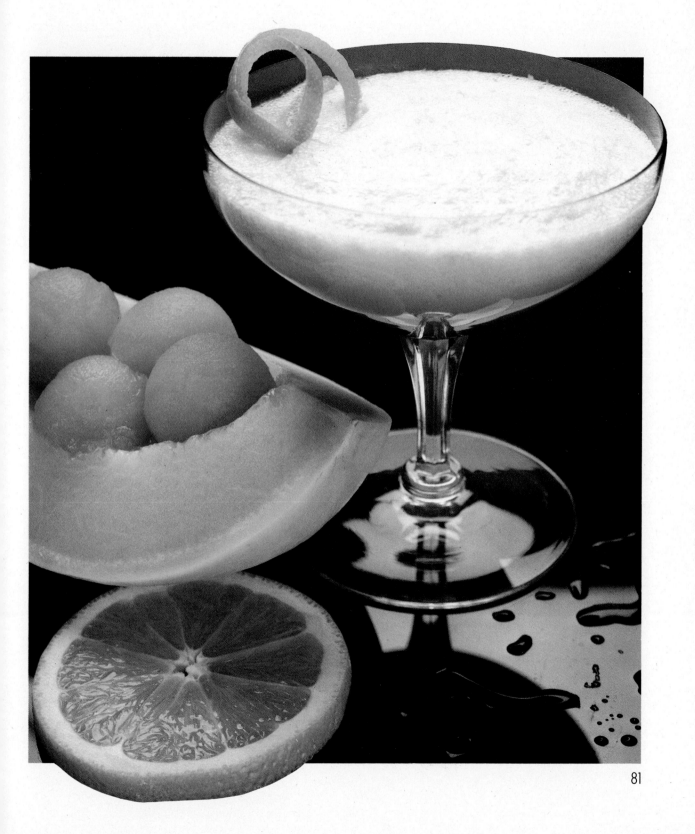

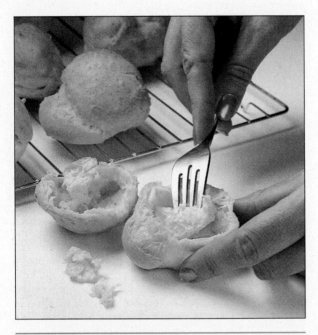

▲ MAKING CREAM PUFFS

In a saucepan bring ½ cup *water* and 2 tablespoons *butter or margarine* to boiling. Add ½ cup *all-purpose flour* and ⅛ teaspoon *salt* all at once. Stir vigorously. Cook and stir till mixture forms a ball that doesn't separate. Remove saucepan from heat and cool for 10 minutes. Add 2 *eggs*, one at a time, beating till smooth after each addition.

Drop mixture by heaping tablespoonfuls into 8 portions 3 inches apart on a lightly greased baking sheet. Bake cream puffs in a 400° oven about 30 minutes or till golden brown and puffy. Remove cream puffs from oven and cut off the tops. Remove the soft centers with a fork as shown, leaving a crisp, hollow puff. Cool on rack. Freeze cream puffs in a tightly covered container to store. Makes 8 cream puffs. (Each unfilled puff provides 74 calories.)

129 APRICOT-PEACH-FILLED PUFFS
Pictured on pages 70 and 71—

4 **Cream Puffs (see tip at left)**
2 **teaspoons cornstarch**
⅛ **teaspoon ground mace *or* ground nutmeg**
⅔ **cup apricot nectar**
¼ **teaspoon finely shredded lemon peel**
2 **medium peaches, peeled, pitted, and coarsely chopped (about 1⅓ cups)**
½ **teaspoon vanilla**

Prepare and bake Cream Puffs. Set the Cream Puffs aside to cool. In a small saucepan combine the cornstarch and the ground mace or ground nutmeg. Stir in the apricot nectar and lemon peel. Cook and stir till mixture is thickened and bubbly. Cook and stir 2 minutes more. Stir peaches and vanilla into apricot mixture. Cover surface with waxed paper; chill. When ready to serve, spoon the apricot-peach mixture into the Cream Puffs. Makes 4 servings.

128 COFFEE-CREAM-FILLED PUFFS
Pictured on pages 70 and 71—

4 **Cream Puffs (see tip at left)**
1 **egg white**
1 **teaspoon instant coffee crystals**
⅛ **teaspoon cream of tartar**
½ **of a 4-ounce container frozen whipped dessert topping, thawed**

Prepare and bake Cream Puffs. Set the Cream Puffs aside to cool. In a small bowl combine the egg white, instant coffee crystals, and cream of tartar, stirring to dissolve the coffee; beat till soft peaks form. Fold in the thawed dessert topping. Cover and chill coffee mixture if desired. Spoon mixture into the Cream Puffs. Makes 4 servings.

DINING OUT POINTERS

- Remember that you don't have to clean your plate. Avoid calories by eating around the breading, fat, gravy, and stuffing.
- If you order a steak, trim fat from meat and cut off the portion of meat you intend to eat. Take the rest home.
- Don't eat the bread and butter that accompany the soup and salad courses.
- Ask for vinegar and oil to dress your salad. Go easy on calorie-laden oil.

115 STRAWBERRY-FLAVORED YOGURT

Next time prepare recipe with fresh or unsweetened frozen raspberries. The homemade yogurt breaks down much easier than the commercial product, so use a minimum amount of stirring—

- 2 8-ounce cartons plain low-fat yogurt or 1¾ cups Homemade Low-Fat Yogurt
- 2 tablespoons sugar
- ½ cup strawberries

Combine yogurt and sugar. Crush berries; gently fold into yogurt. Spoon into dishes. Garnish with a whole berry, if desired. Makes 3 servings.

Homemade Low-Fat Yogurt: In a saucepan heat 2 cups *skim milk* to just below boiling point (200° F), stirring to prevent scorching. Cool to about 115° F, checking temperature with candy thermometer. Place ¼ cup plain low-fat *yogurt* in a bowl; blend in warm milk. Cover bowl with plastic wrap and towel, and place it in another bowl of warm water (115° to 120° F). Let stand 8 to 10 hours or till mixture is firm when shaken gently. Change water every hour to maintain temperature. Let stand 4 hours more to develop tangy flavor. Chill thoroughly. Reserve ¼ cup yogurt to use as a starter for the next batch. Store yogurt and starter in refrigerator. Makes 1¾ cups.

(Note: When you use commercial yogurt as the starter, the first batch of yogurt you make may not set up as firmly as future batches made with your homemade starter. You can discard the free liquid that forms as the yogurt sets up.)

91 LEMON-BLUEBERRY FLUFF

- 1 3-ounce package lemon-flavored gelatin
- ¼ teaspoon finely shredded lemon peel
- 1 tablespoon lemon juice
- 1 egg white
- 1 cup fresh or frozen unsweetened blueberries, thawed
- 2 tablespoons sugar
- 1 tablespoon cornstarch
  Few drops vanilla

In small mixer bowl dissolve gelatin in 1 cup *boiling water*. Stir in lemon peel, lemon juice, and ½ cup *cold water*. Chill till partially set. Add unbeaten egg white to gelatin mixture. Beat with electric mixer 1 to 2 minutes or till mixture is light and fluffy. Pour into six 6-ounce custard cups. Chill till firm. (Slight separation of layers will occur.)

Meanwhile, crush ½ cup of the blueberries. In a small saucepan combine sugar, cornstarch, and ½ cup *cold water*. Add the crushed blueberries. Cook and stir till thickened and bubbly; cook and stir 2 minutes more. Remove from heat; stir in remaining blueberries and vanilla. Chill. To serve, unmold lemon fluff into six individual dessert dishes. Spoon a little blueberry sauce over each dessert. Makes 6 servings.

129 STRAWBERRY CHEESE CREPES

Pictured on pages 70 and 71—

- 6 Calorie Counter's Crepes (see tip, page 55)
- 3 ounces Neufchâtel cheese
- 1 8-ounce carton low-fat strawberry yogurt
- 4 ounces fresh strawberries, sliced (about ½ cup)
- 2 tablespoons powdered sugar

Prepare Calorie Counter's Crepes; set aside. Beat Neufchâtel cheese till fluffy; gradually blend in the yogurt. Fold in the sliced strawberries. Spoon about ⅓ cup of the strawberry mixture along center of unbrowned side of each crepe; fold two opposite sides over. To serve, place one filled crepe on each dessert plate. Sift powdered sugar lightly over top. Makes 6 servings.

24 ZUCCHINI DIP

Calorie count is per tablespoon of dip—

2 medium zucchini, chopped (2 cups)
½ cup tomato juice
1 tablespoon chopped onion
¼ teaspoon salt
⅛ teaspoon dried basil, crushed
1 8-ounce package Neufchâtel cheese, cut up
½ slice bacon, crisp-cooked, drained, and crumbled (optional)

In a saucepan combine the zucchini, tomato juice, onion, salt, and basil. Simmer, covered, for 10 minutes. Turn mixture into blender container. Add the cheese. Cover and blend till mixture is thoroughly combined. Remove from blender. Cover and chill. If desired, just before serving sprinkle top with crumbled bacon. Serve with vegetable dippers. Makes 1¾ cups dip.

76 TACO POPCORN SNACK

2 tablespoons unpopped popcorn (about 2½ cups popped)
1 cup bite-size shredded wheat biscuits
¾ cup round toasted oat cereal
2 tablespoons butter or margarine, melted
½ teaspoon chili powder
⅛ teaspoon onion salt
⅛ teaspoon ground cumin

Pop the popcorn in a heavy skillet or saucepan over medium-high heat using no oil. Be sure to cover pan and shake constantly until all the corn is popped. (Or, pop corn in the microwave oven or popcorn popper following manufacturer's directions.) Combine the popped corn and cereals in a 13x9x2-inch baking pan. Heat in a 300° oven about 5 minutes or till the cereal is warm. Remove from oven. Combine the melted butter or margarine, chili powder, onion salt, and cumin; drizzle over cereal mixture, mixing well. Makes about 8 (½-cup) servings.

16 DILLY COTTAGE DIP

Calorie count is per tablespoon of dip. The dip is pictured on pages 70 and 71—

1 cup low-fat cottage cheese
1 tablespoon mayonnaise or salad dressing
2 tablespoons finely chopped dill pickle
1 tablespoon chopped pimiento
1 tablespoon snipped chives
Skim milk

In a mixing bowl beat together the cottage cheese and mayonnaise. Stir in the dill pickle, pimiento, and chives. If necessary, add enough skim milk to achieve dipping consistency. Serve with vegetable dippers. Makes 1¼ cups dip.

15 TUNA BALLS

Calorie count is for one tuna ball—

1 6½-ounce can tuna (water pack), drained and flaked
1 8-ounce package Neufchâtel cheese
2 tablespoons finely chopped celery
1 teaspoon lemon juice
½ teaspoon Worcestershire sauce
¼ teaspoon salt
⅓ cup finely snipped parsley

In a bowl combine tuna and cheese. Add celery, lemon juice, Worcestershire, and salt; mix well. Chill about 3 hours. Allowing 1½ teaspoons for each, form mixture into balls. Roll in parsley. Chill. To serve, arrange on plate. Makes about 56 balls.

► This assortment of calorie-trimmed foods should please any dieter. Choose from Taco Popcorn Snack, Zucchini Dip, Pickled Shrimp (see recipe, page 86), and Apple-Cot Cooler (see recipe, page 87).

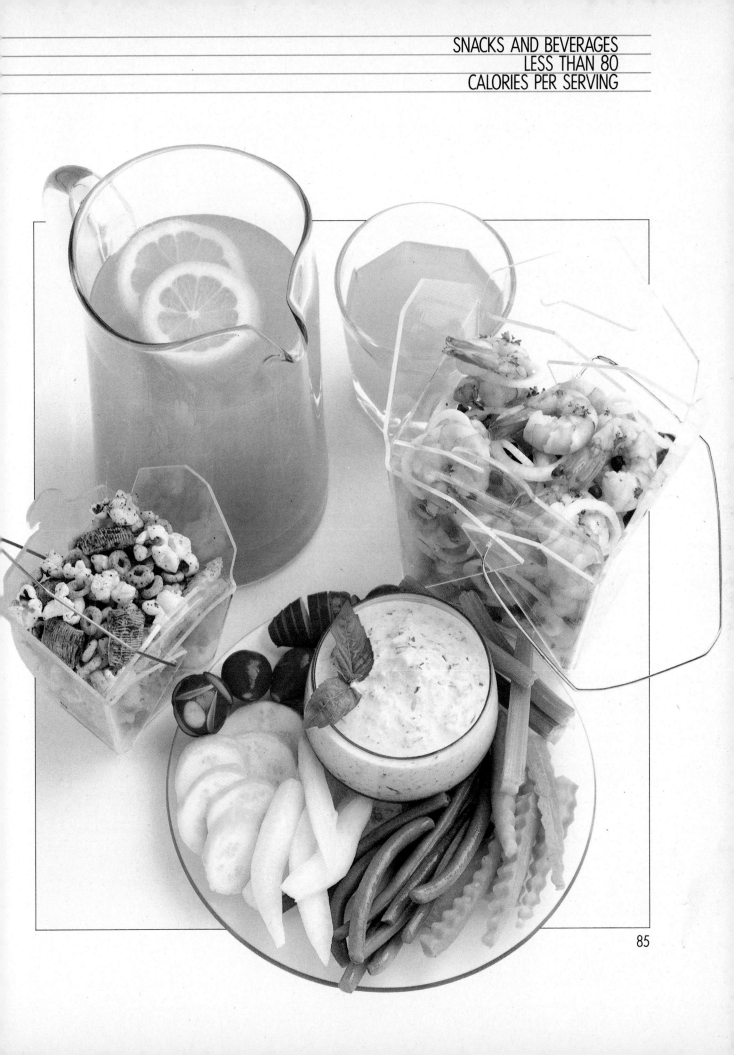

12 ZESTY VEGETABLE DIP

Calorie count is per tablespoon of dip—

1 **10-ounce package frozen peas**
½ **cup chopped onion**
1 **8¾-ounce can whole kernel corn, drained**
½ **teaspoon dried oregano, crushed**
¼ **teaspoon garlic salt**
 Dash bottled hot pepper sauce
½ **cup dairy sour cream**
½ **cup plain low-fat yogurt**
1 **4-ounce can green chili peppers, rinsed, seeded, and chopped**

In a saucepan combine peas, onion, and ½ cup *water*. Bring to boiling. Reduce heat; cover and cook about 5 minutes. Drain, reserving ⅓ cup cooking liquid. In a blender container or food processor bowl combine the cooked vegetables, the reserved liquid, drained corn, oregano, garlic salt, and hot pepper sauce. Cover; process till smooth, scraping sides as necessary. Stir in sour cream, yogurt, and chili peppers. Cover and chill. Garnish dip with pimiento if desired. Serve with assorted dippers such as broccoli flowerets, cauliflower flowerets, zucchini slices, carrot sticks, *or* melba toast rounds. Makes 3½ cups dip.

46 COTTAGE CHEESE-DEVILED EGGS

6 **hard-cooked eggs**
¼ **cup low-fat cottage cheese, drained**
1 **tablespoon snipped parsley**
1 **tablespoon skim milk**
1 **teaspoon vinegar**
1 **teaspoon prepared mustard**
¼ **teaspoon prepared horseradish**
 Snipped parsley (optional)

Halve eggs lengthwise; remove yolks. Set whites aside. In a blender container combine egg yolks, cottage cheese, 1 tablespoon parsley, milk, vinegar, mustard, horseradish, ¼ teaspoon *salt*, and dash *pepper*. Cover; blend till smooth. Stop blender and scrape sides occasionally. Spoon yolk mixture into egg whites; garnish with snipped parsley if desired. Makes 12 egg halves.

60 PICKLED SHRIMP

Pictured on page 85—

2 **tablespoons mixed pickling spices**
3 **cups water**
1 **pound fresh *or* frozen medium shrimp, shelled and deveined**
1 **medium onion, sliced**
½ **cup white wine vinegar**
½ **cup water**
1 **tablespoon capers**
1 **tablespoon snipped parsley**
1 **teaspoon sugar**
½ **teaspoon celery seed**
¼ **teaspoon salt**
¼ **teaspoon dry mustard**
1 **clove garlic, minced**
 Few drops bottled hot pepper sauce

Tie pickling spices in cheesecloth bag. Heat 3 cups water to boiling. Add shrimp, onion, and pickling spices. Return to boiling. Cover and simmer 1 to 3 minutes or till shrimp turn pink. Drain. Place shrimp, onion, and spice bag in a plastic bag set in a deep bowl. Combine the vinegar, ½ cup water, capers with liquid, parsley, sugar, celery seed, salt, dry mustard, garlic, and hot pepper sauce; mix well. Pour mixture over shrimp in bag. Close bag. Marinate in refrigerator at least 24 hours, turning bag occasionally. Serve shrimp with wooden picks. Makes 8 appetizer servings.

VEGETABLE DIPPERS

Use low-calorie raw vegetables for dipping into calorie-counted dips. Suggestions and their approximate calorie counts include:

8 carrot sticks (2½-inch)	**= 12 calories**
3 celery stalks (5-inch)	**= 9 calories**
½ cup green pepper strips	**= 11 calories**
8 small cucumber slices	**= 4 calories**
½ cup cauliflower flowerets	**= 14 calories**
½ cup mushroom slices	**= 10 calories**
10 medium radishes	**= 8 calories**

67 STRAWBERRY SHAKE

2 cups fresh *or* frozen whole strawberries
1½ cups skim milk
2 tablespoons sugar
Dash ground cinnamon

If you are using fresh strawberries, halve large berries. Freeze berries. In a blender container combine the skim milk, sugar, and ground cinnamon; gradually add the frozen berries, blending at medium speed till smooth. Serve immediately in small glasses. Makes 5 (5-ounce) servings.

67 HOT FRUITY SPICED TEA

1 18-ounce can (2¼ cups) unsweetened pineapple juice
2 cups orange juice
2 tablespoons instant tea powder
1 teaspoon whole allspice
3 inches stick cinnamon, broken up

In a saucepan mix 2 cups *water*, the pineapple juice, orange juice, tea powder, and spices. Bring to boiling; reduce heat. Simmer, covered, for 15 minutes. Strain or use a slotted spoon to remove spices. Serve hot. Makes 8 (6-ounce) servings.

60 APPLE-COT COOLER

Pictured on page 85—

2 cups apple juice
1 12-ounce can apricot nectar
¼ cup lemon juice
¼ teaspoon aromatic bitters
2 cups carbonated water, chilled
8 thin lemon slices

Combine apple juice, nectar, lemon juice, and bitters; chill. Before serving, carefully pour carbonated water down side of pitcher. Stir gently with an up-and-down motion. Serve over ice. Garnish with lemon. Makes 8 (6-ounce) servings.

71 FRUIT SLUSH

Pictured on pages 70 and 71—

2 16-ounce bottles low-calorie lemon-lime carbonated beverage
1 6-ounce can frozen lemonade concentrate, limeade concentrate, orange juice concentrate, *or* pineapple-orange juice concentrate, thawed

Pour the low-calorie lemon-lime carbonated beverage into an 8x8x2-inch pan; freeze till firm. Break frozen carbonated beverage into chunks and crush. Pour the desired thawed fruit concentrate into a blender container; add the frozen crushed beverage to the blender container, 1 cup at a time, blending well after each addition. Stop blender several times and push ice down from sides. Spoon the mixture into six glasses. Garnish each serving with fresh fruit if desired. Makes 6 (6-ounce) servings.

79 BREAKFAST MOCHA COCOA

Pictured in the breakfast menu on page 13—

2 tablespoons unsweetened cocoa powder
1 tablespoon sugar
2 teaspoons instant coffee crystals
2¾ cups skim milk
3 inches stick cinnamon
Cinnamon stick stirrers (optional)

In a saucepan mix the unsweetened cocoa powder, sugar, and instant coffee crystals. Add the skim milk and 3 inches stick cinnamon. Heat just till hot but *do not boil.* Remove from heat. Remove the stick cinnamon piece. Beat mixture with a rotary beater till frothy. Pour into four mugs. If desired, garnish with additional cinnamon stick stirrers. Makes 4 servings.

CALORIE CHART

A-B

- **ANCHOVIES,** canned; 5 fillets 35
- **APPLE BUTTER;** 1 tablespoon 33
- **APPLES**
  fresh; 1 medium.. 80
  juice, canned; 1 cup 117
- **APPLESAUCE,** canned
  sweetened; ½ cup.. 116
  unsweetened; ½ cup..................................... 50
- **APRICOTS**
  canned, in syrup; ½ cup 111
  dried, cooked, unsweetened, in juice; ½ cup....... 106
  fresh; 3 medium.. 55
  nectar, canned; 1 cup 143
- **ASPARAGUS**
  cooked, drained; 4 medium spears 12
  cooked, drained; ½ cup cut............................ 15
- **AVOCADO,** peeled; ½ avocado........................ 188
- **BACON**
  Canadian-style, cooked; 1 slice 58
  crisp strips, medium thickness; 2...................... 86
- **BANANA;** 1 medium 101
- **BARBECUE SAUCE,** bottled; ½ cup 114
- **BEANS**
  baked, with tomato sauce and pork, canned;
    ½ cup 155
  green snap, cooked; ½ cup.............................. 16
  lima, cooked; ½ cup...................................... 95
  red kidney, canned; ½ cup 115
  yellow or wax, cooked; ½ cup 14
- **BEAN SPROUTS,** fresh; ½ cup 18
- **BEEF,** dried, chipped; 2 ounces...................... 116
- **BEEF CUTS**
  corned, canned; 3 ounces 184
  ground beef, cooked, 21% fat; 3 ounces............. 243
  ground beef, cooked, 10% fat; 3 ounces............. 186
  pot roast, cooked, lean and fat; 3 ounces........... 246
  pot roast, cooked, lean only; 3 ounces 164
  rib roast, cooked, lean and fat; 3 ounces 374
  rib roast, cooked, lean only; 3 ounces 205
  round steak, cooked, lean only; 3 ounces........... 161
  sirloin steak, broiled, lean and fat; 3 ounces........ 329
- **BEEF LIVER,** fried; 2 ounces 130
- **BEETS,** cooked, diced; ½ cup 27
- **BEVERAGES,** alcoholic
  beer; 1 cup.. 101
  dessert wine; 1 ounce.................................... 41
  gin, rum, vodka—80 proof; 1 jigger.................... 97
  table wine; 1 ounce....................................... 25

- **BISCUIT,** baking powder;
    1 (2-inch diameter) 103
- **BLACKBERRIES,** fresh; ½ cup 42
- **BLUEBERRIES**
  fresh; ½ cup 45
  frozen, sweetened; ½ cup 121
- **BOUILLON,** instant granules; 1 teaspoon............... 2
- **BOYSENBERRIES,** frozen, unsweetened;
    ½ cup 30
- **BREAD**
  Boston brown; 1 slice (3¼x½ inches)................. 95
  breadstick, plain; 1 (7¾ inches long)................. 19
  bun, frankfurter or hamburger; 1...................... 119
  corn bread; 1 piece (2½x2½x1½ inches)........... 161
  crumbs, dry; ¼ cup...................................... 98
  crumbs, soft; ¼ cup...................................... 30
  cubes; 1 cup.. 81
  French; 1 slice (½ inch thick) 44
  Italian; 1 slice (½ inch thick) 28
  pumpernickel; 1 slice 79
  raisin; 1 slice 66
  rye; 1 slice.. 61
  white; 1 slice 68
  whole wheat; 1 slice 56
- **BROCCOLI**
  cooked; 1 medium stalk................................. 47
  frozen chopped, cooked; ½ cup 24
- **BRUSSELS SPROUTS,** cooked; ½ cup.............. 28
- **BUTTER**
  1 pat (about 1 teaspoon)................................ 36
  1 tablespoon 102

C

- **CABBAGE**
  Chinese, raw; ½ cup 1-inch pieces 6
  common varieties, raw, shredded; 1 cup 17
  red, raw, shredded; 1 cup............................... 22
- **CAKE,** baked from home recipes
  angel, no icing; 1/12 cake 161
  chocolate, 2 layers, chocolate icing;
    2-inch wedge 365
  fruitcake; 1 slice (2x1½x¼ inches) 57
  gingerbread; 1 piece (3x3x2 inches) 371
  pound; 1 slice (3½x3x½ inches) 142
  sponge, no icing; 1/12 cake 131
  white, uncooked white icing; 1/12 cake.............. 390
  yellow, chocolate icing; 1/12 cake 365
- **CANDY**
  caramel; 1 ounce (3 medium) 113
  chocolate bar, milk; 1 ounce 147
  chocolate fudge; 1 piece (1 cubic inch) 84
  gumdrops; 1 ounce 98
  hard; 1 ounce.. 109

► **EGG**
fried; 1 large 99
poached, hard- or soft-cooked; 1 medium 72
scrambled, plain; made with 1 large egg 111
whole; 1 large 82
whole; 1 medium 72
► **EGGPLANT,** cooked, diced; ½ cup 19
► **ENDIVE,** raw; 1 cup 10
► **FIGS**
canned, in syrup; ½ cup 109
dried; 1 large 52
raw; 3 small 96
► **FISH**
bass, baked; 3 ounces 219
flounder, baked; 3 ounces 171
haddock, fried; 3 ounces 141
halibut, broiled; 3 ounces 144
herring, pickled; 3 ounces 189
ocean perch, fried; 3 ounces 192
salmon, broiled or baked; 3 ounces 156
salmon, canned, pink; ½ cup 155
sardines, canned, in oil, drained; 3 ounces 174
swordfish, broiled; 3 ounces 138
tuna, canned, in oil, drained; ½ cup 158
tuna, canned, in water, drained; ½ cup 126
► **FISH STICK,** breaded; 1 50
► **FLOUR,** wheat
all-purpose; 1 cup 455
whole wheat; 1 cup 400
► **FRANKFURTER,** cooked; 1 139
► **FRUIT COCKTAIL**
canned, in syrup; ½ cup 97
canned, water-pack; ½ cup 45
► **GARBANZO BEANS,** cooked; ½ cup 129
► **GARLIC,** peeled; 1 clove 4
► **GELATIN,** dry, unflavored; 1 envelope 23
► **GELATIN DESSERT,** plain, ready-to-serve;
½ cup 71
► **GINGER ALE;** 1 cup 72
► **GOOSE,** cooked; 3 ounces 198
► **GOOSEBERRIES,** raw; 1 cup 59
► **GRAPEFRUIT**
canned sections, in syrup; ½ cup 89
fresh; ½ medium 40
juice, canned, sweetened; 1 cup 133
juice, canned, unsweetened; 1 cup 101
juice, fresh; 1 cup 96
juice, frozen, sweetened, reconstituted; 1 cup 117
juice, frozen, unsweetened, reconstituted;
1 cup 101

► **GRAPES**
concord, fresh; ½ cup 35
green, fresh, seedless; ½ cup 54
juice, canned; 1 cup 167

H-O

► **HAM,** fully cooked, lean only; 3 ounces 159
► **HONEY;** 1 tablespoon 64
► **HONEYDEW MELON;** ¼ medium (6½-inch
diameter) 124
► **HORSERADISH,** prepared; 1 tablespoon 6
► **ICE CREAM,** vanilla
ice milk; 1 cup 199
soft-serve; 1 cup 266
10% fat; 1 cup 257
► **JAM;** 1 tablespoon 54
► **JELLY;** 1 tablespoon 49
► **KALE,** cooked; ½ cup 22
► **KOHLRABI,** cooked, diced; ½ cup 20
► **LAMB,** cooked
loin chop, lean only; 3 ounces 160
rib chop, lean only; 3 ounces 179
roast leg, lean only; 3 ounces 158
► **LARD;** 1 tablespoon 117
► **LEMON;** 1 medium 20
► **LEMONADE,** frozen, sweetened, reconstituted;
1 cup 107
► **LEMON JUICE;** 1 tablespoon 4
► **LENTILS,** cooked; ½ cup 106
► **LETTUCE**
Boston; ¼ medium head 6
iceberg, ¼ medium compact head 18
iceberg, 1 leaf (5x4½ inches) 3
► **LIME;** 1 medium 19
► **LIMEADE,** frozen, sweetened, reconstituted;
1 cup 102
► **LIME JUICE;** 1 tablespoon 4
► **LIVERWURST;** 2 ounces 174
► **LOBSTER,** cooked; ½ cup 69
► **LUNCHEON MEAT**
bologna; 1 ounce 86
ham, boiled; 1 ounce 66
salami, cooked; 1 ounce 88
► **MACARONI,** cooked; ½ cup 78
► **MALTED MILK;** 1 cup 244
► **MAPLE SYRUP;** 1 tablespoon 50
► **MARGARINE;** 1 tablespoon 102
► **MARSHMALLOWS;** 1 ounce 90
► **MELBA TOAST;** 1 slice 15
► **MILK**
buttermilk; 1 cup 88
chocolate drink (2% fat); 1 cup 190
condensed, sweetened, undiluted; 1 cup 982

MILK (continued)
dried nonfat, instant, reconstituted; 1 cup 81
evaporated, undiluted; 1 cup 345
low-fat (2% fat); 1 cup 145
skim; 1 cup 88
whole; 1 cup... 159
▶ **MOLASSES,** light; 1 tablespoon 50
▶ **MUFFIN**
blueberry; 1... 112
bran; 1 104
plain; 1 118
▶ **MUSHROOMS,** raw; 1 cup 20
▶ **MUSTARD,** prepared; 1 tablespoon...................... 12
▶ **MUSTARD GREENS,** cooked; ½ cup 16
▶ **NECTARINE,** fresh; 1 (2½-inch diameter)............. 88
▶ **NOODLES,** chow mein, canned; 1 cup 220
▶ **NOODLES**
cooked; ½ cup... 100
dry; 1 ounce 110
▶ **NUTS**
almonds, shelled, chopped; 1 tablespoon.............. 48
Brazil nuts; 3 89
cashews, roasted; 1 ounce 159
peanuts, roasted, shelled, chopped;
  1 tablespoon.. 52
pecans, chopped; 1 tablespoon 52
pistachio; 1 ounce 168
walnuts, chopped; 1 tablespoon......................... 52
▶ **OIL,** corn; 1 tablespoon 120
▶ **OKRA**
fresh, cooked; 10 pods (3x⅝ inches) 31
frozen, cooked; ½ cup 35
▶ **OLIVES,** green; 4 medium 15
▶ **OLIVES,** ripe; 3 small 15
▶ **ONIONS**
cooked; ½ cup.. 30
green, without tops; 6 small................................ 14
mature, raw, chopped; 1 tablespoon 4
▶ **ORANGES**
fresh; 1 medium... 64
juice, canned, unsweetened; 1 cup 120
juice, fresh; 1 cup 112
juice, frozen concentrate, reconstituted; 1 cup 122
▶ **OYSTERS**
fried; 1 ounce 68
raw; ½ cup (6 to 10 medium) 79

P-S

▶ **PANCAKES;** 1 (4-inch diameter) 62
▶ **PAPAYA;** 1.. 119
▶ **PARSLEY,** raw; 1 tablespoon................................ 2

▶ **PARSNIPS,** cooked, diced; ½ cup 51
▶ **PEACHES**
canned, in syrup; 1 half and 2 tablespoons
  syrup 75
canned, water-pack; ½ cup 38
fresh; 1 medium... 38
frozen, sweetened; ½ cup 110
▶ **PEANUT BUTTER;** 1 tablespoon 94
▶ **PEARS**
canned, in syrup; 1 half and 2 tablespoons
  syrup 71
fresh; 1 medium... 100
▶ **PEAS,** green, cooked; ½ cup 57
▶ **PEPPER,** green, sweet, chopped; ½ cup 16
▶ **PICKLE RELISH,** sweet; 1 tablespoon................. 21
▶ **PICKLES**
dill; 1 large (4x1¾ inches) 15
sweet; 1 medium (2¾x¾ inches)......................... 30
▶ **PIE,** ⅛ of a 9-inch pie
apple.. 302
blueberry.. 286
cherry 308
custard 249
lemon meringue... 268
pumpkin 241
▶ **PIE SHELL,** baked; one 9-inch 900
▶ **PIMIENTO;** 2 tablespoons 7
▶ **PINEAPPLE**
canned, in syrup; ½ cup................................... 95
canned, water-pack; ½ cup 48
fresh, diced; ½ cup 40
juice, canned, unsweetened; 1 cup 138
▶ **PLUMS**
canned, syrup-pack; ½ cup 107
fresh; 1 (2-inch diameter) 32
▶ **POPCORN,** plain, popped; 1 cup......................... 23
▶ **PORK,** cooked
chop, loin center cut, lean only; 3 ounces 226
picnic shoulder, fresh, lean only; 3 ounces.......... 180
sausage, links or patty; 3 ounces 291
▶ **POTATO CHIPS;** 10 medium 114
▶ **POTATOES**
baked; 1 medium (oblong) 145
boiled; 1 medium (round).................................... 104
french fried, frozen, oven heated; 10 medium 172
french fried, homemade; 10 medium 214
hash brown; ½ cup 177
mashed with milk; ½ cup................................... 68
scalloped and au gratin, with cheese; ½ cup....... 178
scalloped and au gratin, without cheese;
  ½ cup 128
sweet, baked; 1 medium.................................... 161
sweet, canned, vacuum packed; ½ cup 108

▶ **POTATO STICKS;** 1 cup 190
▶ **PRETZELS;** 10 small sticks 23
▶ **PRUNE JUICE,** canned; 1 cup 197
▶ **PRUNES,** dried
  cooked, unsweetened; ½ cup 127
  uncooked, pitted; 1 cup 459
▶ **PUDDING,** cornstarch
  chocolate; ½ cup 193
  vanilla; ½ cup 142
▶ **PUMPKIN,** canned; 1 cup 81
▶ **RABBIT,** domestic, cooked; 3 ounces 185
▶ **RADISHES,** raw; 5 medium 4
▶ **RAISINS;** 1 cup 419
▶ **RASPBERRIES**
  black, fresh; ½ cup 49
  red, fresh; ½ cup 35
  red, frozen, sweetened; ½ cup 122
▶ **RHUBARB**
  cooked, sweetened; ½ cup 191
  raw, diced; 1 cup 20
▶ **RICE**
  brown, cooked; ½ cup 116
  white, cooked; ½ cup 112
  white, quick-cooking, cooked; ½ cup 90
▶ **ROLL**
  cloverleaf; 1 (2½-inch diameter) 119
  hard; 1 medium 156
  hard; 1 small 78
  sweet; 1 medium 274
▶ **RUSK;** 1 (3⅜-inch diameter, ½ inch thick) 38
▶ **RUTABAGAS,** cooked, cubed; ½ cup 30
▶ **SALAD DRESSING**
  blue cheese; 1 tablespoon 76
  French; 1 tablespoon 66
  Italian; 1 tablespoon 83
  mayonnaise; 1 tablespoon 101
  mayonnaise-type; 1 tablespoon 65
  Russian; 1 tablespoon 74
  Thousand Island; 1 tablespoon 80
▶ **SAUERKRAUT,** canned; ½ cup 21
▶ **SCALLOPS,** cooked; 3 ounces 95
▶ **SHERBET,** orange; ½ cup 130
▶ **SHORTENING;** 1 tablespoon 111
▶ **SHRIMP**
  canned; 3 ounces 100
  French fried; 3 ounces 192
▶ **SOUP,** condensed, canned, diluted with water
   unless specified otherwise
  beef bouillon, broth, consommé; 1 cup 31
  beef noodle; 1 cup 67
  chicken noodle; 1 cup 62
  clam chowder, Manhattan-style; 1 cup 81
  cream of celery, diluted with milk; 1 cup 169

▶ **SOUP** (continued)
  cream of mushroom, diluted with milk; 1 cup 216
  split pea; 1 cup 145
  tomato; 1 cup 88
  tomato, diluted with milk; 1 cup 173
  vegetable with beef broth; 1 cup 78
▶ **SOUR CREAM,** dairy; ½ cup 247
▶ **SOY SAUCE;** 1 tablespoon 12
▶ **SPAGHETTI,** cooked, plain; ½ cup 78
▶ **SPINACH**
  canned; ½ cup 22
  frozen, chopped, cooked; ½ cup 25
  raw, torn; 1 cup 14
▶ **SQUASH**
  summer, cooked, diced; ½ cup 15
  winter, baked, mashed; ½ cup 65
▶ **STRAWBERRIES**
  fresh, whole; ½ cup 28
  frozen, sweetened, whole; ½ cup 117
▶ **SUCCOTASH,** frozen, cooked; ½ cup 79
▶ **SUGAR**
  brown, packed; 1 tablespoon 51
  granulated; 1 tablespoon 46
  powdered; 1 tablespoon 31

T-Z

▶ **TANGERINE;** 1 medium 39
▶ **TARTAR SAUCE;** 1 tablespoon 74
▶ **TEA** 0
▶ **TOFU** (soybean curd); 1 pound 327
▶ **TOMATOES**
  canned; ½ cup 25
  fresh; 1 medium 27
  juice, canned; 1 cup 46
  paste, canned; 6 ounces 139
  sauce; 1 cup 70
▶ **TURKEY,** roasted; 3 slices (3 ounces) 162
▶ **TURNIP GREENS,** cooked; ½ cup 15
▶ **TURNIPS,** cooked, diced; ½ cup 18
▶ **VEAL,** cooked
  cutlet; 3 ounces 184
  loin chop; 3 ounces 199
▶ **VEGETABLE JUICE COCKTAIL;** 1 cup 41
▶ **VINEGAR;** 1 tablespoon 2
▶ **WAFFLE;** 1 section (4½x4½x⅝ inches) 140
▶ **WATERCRESS,** raw, chopped; ½ cup 12
▶ **WATERMELON;** 1 wedge (8x4 inches) 111
▶ **YOGURT**
  low-fat fruit-flavored; ½ cup 115
  plain, made from skim milk; ½ cup 61
  plain, made from whole milk; ½ cup 76
▶ **ZWIEBACK;** 1 piece 30

INDEX

93